HELP IS HERE!

Treat Your PMS Symptoms with Food for the Complete Health of Your Body and Soul

Do you suffer from . . .

Cramps? Try Roasted Chicken with Kasha and Wild M

Mood swings? Try Vegetable Paella Primer or Fresh

Intense sugar cravings? Try Chunky Vegetable Minestrone with Cannellini Beans

Beat fatigue with Silky Peach Custard with Pistachios and Cardamom Swirl

Alleviate depression and anxiety with Mushroom Bouquet Soup with Wild Rice

Relieve swollen, tender breasts with Sweet Potato and Turnip Stew with Chicken Strips

Reduce irritability with Creamy Hungarian Asparagus Soup or Sesame Lemon Snaps with Almonds or French Leek, Broccoli, and Potato Quiche

Ease feelings of bloating with Broccoli Salad with Red Onion and Black Olives

. . . and more

Lissa G. De Angelis is a nutritionist with a master of science in Human Nutrition and certified as a chef and culinary professional. She is the former associate director of the Natural Gourmet Cookery School in New York and has worked in the field of natural healing and nutrition since 1972. She writes nutrition and cooking columns for several magazines, maintains an active lecture and teaching schedule, and has a nutritional consulting business. She can be contacted at *LDeAngelis@aol.com*.

Molly Siple is a registered dietitian with a master of science in Nutrition. She lectures and consults on diet and wellness in Los Angeles, and writes a monthly newsletter about women's health on her website: *www.wellwoman.com*.

ALSO BY THE AUTHORS

*Recipes for Change: Gourmet Wholefood Cooking for
Health and Vitality at Menopause*

SOS *for* PMS

Whole-Food Solutions for Premenstrual Syndrome

Lissa G. De Angelis and Molly Siple

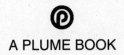

A PLUME BOOK

W

A NOTE TO THE READER: The ideas, procedures, and suggestions contained in this book are not intended as a substitute for consulting with your physician. All matters regarding your health require medical supervision.

PLUME
Published by the Penguin Group
Penguin Putnam Inc., 375 Hudson Street, New York, New York 10014, U.S.A.
Penguin Books Ltd, 27 Wrights Lane, London W8 5TZ, England
Penguin Books Australia Ltd, Ringwood, Victoria, Australia
Penguin Books Canada Ltd, 10 Alcorn Avenue, Toronto, Ontario, Canada M4V 3B2
Penguin Books (N.Z.) Ltd, 182–190 Wairau Road, Auckland 10, New Zealand

Penguin Books Ltd, Registered Offices: Harmondsworth, Middlesex, England

First published by Plume, a member of Penguin Putnam Inc.

First Printing, June, 1999

1 3 5 7 9 10 8 6 4 2

 REGISTERED TRADEMARK—MARCA REGISTRADA

LIBRARY OF CONGRESS CATALOGING-IN-PUBLICATION DATA
De Angelis, Lissa.
SOS for PMS : whole-food solutions for premenstrual syndrome /
Lissa G. De Angelis and Molly Siple.
p.   cm.
Includes bibliographical references and index.
ISBN 0-452-27965-8
1. Premenstrual syndrome—Nutritional aspects—Popular works.
I. Siple, Molly.   II. Title.
RG165.D43   1999
618.1'72—dc21   98-32106
CIP

Printed in the United States of America
Set in Garamond Light and Tiffany
Designed by Eve L. Kirch

BOOKS ARE AVAILABLE AT QUANTITY DISCOUNTS WHEN USED TO PROMOTE PRODUCTS OR SERVICES. FOR INFORMATION PLEASE WRITE TO PREMIUM MARKETING DIVISION, PENGUIN PUTNAM INC., 375 HUDSON STREET, NEW YORK, NEW YORK 10014.

To all women—as we learn about our bodies,
how to care for ourselves,
and how to maintain good health.

ACKNOWLEDGMENTS

Thank you to Victor for organization, Esma for proofreading, Dee for friendship, Susan for inspiration, and Lissa for partnership.—*Molly Siple*

I would like to acknowledge and express my gratitude for the love and support of the following people:

Cosmo—throughout eternity, as we continue together, giving each other the greatest gift there is—love. My thankfulness to you is wordless.

To my father, who in spirit is with me in all ways. Thank you for the gift of freedom.

To my mother, my greatest teacher and friend, who taught me to have faith in myself and to enjoy life.

For Helene, Bob, Joshua, and Kimberly whose generosity of spirit shines through all they touch.

For all the happiness they bring—Victor and Tessie; Lisa, Dawn, and Jennifer; and Jack, Dianna, and family.

To the cheering team for their constant support and encouragement—Linda and Bruce Seiden, Ugo Polla, Chris and Mark Seasly, Bea and Jim Fitzpatrick, Nicholas Gonzalez, M.D., Bob and Joan Axelrod, Ann Nolan, Marie Mattie, and Cathy Bruno.

And many thanks to Annemarie Colbin especially for the introduction to my dear co-author, Molly Siple.—*Lissa De Angelis*

And from the both of us—we thank Carole DeSanti, Alexandra Babanskyj, and the team effort it takes from all of the hardworking and creative staff at Penguin Putnam.

CONTENTS

SOS *for* PMS

Introduction

You have within easy reach a simple and effective way to prevent and treat your symptoms of premenstrual syndrome—food! The vegetables, fruits, grains, meats, and fish that you choose to eat contain vitamins, minerals, and even fats that influence your body chemistry and profoundly affect how you feel throughout the month. Foods that help balance hormones and promote a healthy nervous system initiate processes that can prevent such menstrual symptoms as irritability, fluid retention, and headaches. The way you can benefit from this culinary chemistry is by being aware of which foods are best for you—and then eating them!

The following pages provide an overview of the various symptoms of PMS and their origins, and give you a quick overview of the foods that can come to your rescue. We then explain how various categories of food affect symptoms. A list of the specific nutrients that are especially beneficial for treating PMS, and simple dietary guidelines for each type of PMS follows.

A wonderful assortment of fresh, unrefined, unprocessed foods can help restore normal body chemistry and prevent PMS. The over one hundred easy-to-cook recipes in this book incorporate these foods as ingredients. When you cook the way we recommend with vegetables that are in season and at the peak of their flavor; with fresh, sweet-tasting fish; and with richly flavored unprocessed oils, you'll be enjoying foods that directly support your menstrual health and have proven therapeutic benefits. Such nutritious meals can also be the tastiest!

This text is really two books in one, both a nutrition book and a cookbook. We suggest that before experimenting with the recipes you first read through this introduction and then thumb through the recipe pages, reading the PMS benefits at the beginning of each recipe. This will give you an overview of the way of eating we suggest, and help you to begin eating foods you need, whether you are dining out, grabbing some take-out food, or cooking at home.

Your Monthly Cycle

The menstrual process is one of cleansing. In anticipation of new life, the lining of the uterus thickens and the blood supply to the area increases, preparing to receive a fertilized egg. The ovaries produce many eggs, one of which is expelled to unite with a sperm for conception. If the egg and the sperm fail to unite, the uterus must shed its lining and prepare again to be a home to a developing embryo.

The phases of the menstrual cycle are controlled by hormones. During the first phase, estrogen stimulates the lining of the uterus to thicken. When estrogen levels peak, ovulation occurs. In the next phase, progesterone dominates and is essential for maintaining pregnancy. If pregnancy does not occur, the uterus sheds its lining, which a woman experiences as menstruation. Symptoms relate to these changing hormone levels—for instance, elevated estrogen is associated with anxiety, while progesterone dominance can lead to depression.

Each menstrual cycle lasts approximately twenty-eight days and occurs approximately four hundred and fifty times in a woman's life. The rhythmic changes of hormone levels during the cycle are highly interdependent, as hormones that are produced by glands in one area of the body travel to another, where they signal the production of a different hormone or cause a certain chemical change. The phases of the menstrual cycle depend on one hormone triggering another, and given how hormones interact, any irregularity in this system can bring on symptoms of PMS.

Factors that can increase a woman's risk of developing PMS include fatigue, allergies, food sensitivities, birth-control pills, gynecological disorders such as fibroids or endometriosis, multiple childbirths, and being over thirty. Inefficient liver function may also be a cause of hormonal imbalance. As the body's organ of detoxification, the liver breaks down the toxins the body has been exposed to and absorbed. It also deactivates excess hormones, such as estrogen. However, when the liver is overburdened with toxins, it is less able to manage hormone levels, and you are more likely to feel the ups and downs of PMS. A history of unresolved physical or sexual abuse may also lie at the root of menstrual problems. However, more commonly than not, the lifestyle habits typical of women today, such as lack of exercise, stress, and poor diet, are the most likely reasons that PMS develops.

If You Have PMS, You Have Company!

If you're feeling blue or bloated, you are not alone. Studies conducted around the world suggest that from 40 to 95 percent of women experience PMS to some degree. According to the Madison Women's Pharmacy, which disseminates information on PMS and has worked with over 600,000 women, about 97 percent of women have PMS at some point in their lives. Of these, about 40 percent have symptoms that are intense enough to be troubling. Another 5 percent feel so incapacitated by anxiety, depression, and migraines that they regularly withdraw to their bedroom for a day or two or may even require emergency medical treatment.

PMS regularly strikes women in their thirties and forties, when the most severe symptoms can occur. Symptoms may intensify as a woman approaches menopause, a phase known as perimenopause, when hormone production becomes irregular. Furthermore, the number of young women in their teens and twenties who experience PMS is on the rise. It is well documented that many young women have a poor diet, high in fat and low in fruits and vegetables. In some cases, these women also regularly consume alcohol, smoke, and rarely exercise. Here is an opportunity for mothers of teenage daughters to alleviate menstrual problems by helping their daughters change these habits. Mothers can begin by shopping for foods and preparing meals with health-enhancing ingredients. A bonus of this way of eating is that these foods also support health in many other ways so that cooking more nutritious foods will benefit everyone in the family.

PMS Symptoms

Health professionals and researchers have identified as many as 150 physical and psychological symptoms of PMS—everything from crying spells and sugar cravings to puffiness and clumsiness. Which ones best describe your version of PMS? Following each group of symptoms are some dietary guidelines, your keys to developing menus that can remedy a specific type of PMS. For a more in-depth discussion of particular food groups, as well as vitamins and minerals, you can also refer to the sections that follow and to the Appendix.

Irritability—Anxiety—Mood Swings—Nervous Tension

Chances are if you experience PMS, you're familiar with this annoying group of symptoms, which friends and family may complain about as well! Irritability, anxiety, and associated symptoms can occur when estrogen is elevated in relation to progesterone. Low levels of endorphins, compounds that elevate mood, and dramatic dips in blood sugar also trigger these symptoms. (See the section "Sugars and Sweeteners" on page 11.)

Food choices: herbal teas, fruit juice, filtered water rather than caffeinated drinks; maple syrup or honey; eliminate all refined sugar.

Nutrients: B vitamins—whole grains, fish, blackstrap molasses; vitamin B6—beans, whole grains, meat; magnesium—green vegetables, whole grains, nuts, seafood; zinc—pumpkinseeds, sunflower seeds, mushrooms; flavonoids—black currants, fresh berries, buckwheat, citrus.

Carbohydrate Cravings—Sugar Cravings—Increased Appetite— Fatigue—Dizziness—Shakiness—Fainting—Headaches—Palpitations

Sixty percent of women with PMS crave carbohydrates, such as chocolate cake or cookies. Elevated levels of insulin, five to ten days before menstruation, prompt cells to absorb glucose rapidly, thereby lowering the levels of sugar in the blood. The body attempts to compensate for this drop in blood sugar by developing cravings for sugar and starchy carbohydrates. Your craving for sweets may also be an instinctive attempt to self-medicate menstrual anxiety. When we eat carbohydrates, the body produces more of the neurotransmitter serotonin, which generates a feeling of calmness and well-being. Note that certain medical conditions such as hypothyroidism, chronic fatigue syndrome, and yeast infection may masquerade as this form of PMS. If these health problems are suspected, it is important to seek the care of an informed physician to treat these conditions appropriately.

Food choices: complex carbohydrates such as whole wheat bread rather than refined flour; brown rice and barley rather than refined grains; butter, extra-virgin olive oil rather than refined oils; maple syrup or honey rather than refined sugar.

Nutrients: B vitamins—beans, peas, blackstrap molasses; magnesium—millet, nuts, dark-green vegetables; vitamin E—extra-virgin olive oil, flaxseed oil, kale, organic eggs; omega-3 EFA's (essential fatty acids)—flaxseed oil, salmon and tuna, walnuts; vitamin C, magnesium, zinc, and B vitamins to facilitate use of the EFA's—green peppers, whole grains, oysters, and molasses.

Fluid Retention—Weight Gain—Abdominal Bloating—Swollen Hands and Feet—Breast Tenderness

Approximately 40 percent of women experience these symptoms. To understand their underlying dynamics, you need to keep in mind that salt draws water to it. Your body makes use of this property to control how much fluid is retained and where. Your kidneys maintain sodium and fluid levels, and any hormonal disruption will hamper their ability to excrete sodium and lead to bloating. Elevated amounts of insulin, due to the overconsumption of refined sugar, and a deficiency of vitamin B6 also promote fluid retention.

Food choices: sea salt in moderation rather than commercial table salt; maple syrup or honey; avoid refined sugar.

Nutrients: vitamin B6—whole grains, legumes, green leafy vegetables; magnesium— millet, organic eggs, almonds.

Depression—Crying—Forgetfulness—Confusion—Insomnia

If you are feeling blue, you're most likely experiencing an imbalance of estrogen and progesterone. Estrogen is a mood elevator and progesterone a depressant. An excess of progesterone in relation to estrogen promotes depression and its related symptoms. Low levels of neurotransmitters in the central nervous system can also be a cause, as can unstable blood sugar, which can bring on tears as glucose levels dip.

Food choices: eat regularly scheduled meals, and be sure to include breakfast; avoid refined flour and sugar.

Nutrients: magnesium—buckwheat, eggs, almonds; B-complex vitamins—whole grains such as barley and oats, beans and peas, blackstrap molasses; potassium— vegetables, dried fruits, legumes, whole grains, sunflower seeds; EFA's—fish, organic eggs, vegetables, nuts, seeds.

Oily Scalp and Hair—Pimples—Acne

While women mostly produce female sex hormones, we also produce a small amount of male sex hormones or androgens. Levels of androgens may increase pre-menstrually, and your skin and hair can become oily. Serious skin problems such as severe acne, cold sores, and hives may require medical treatment.

Food choices: refrain from eating nuts, seeds, and very oily foods seven to ten days before your menstrual cycle begins.

Nutrients: potassium—black beans, pinto beans, kelp, potatoes, turkey; zinc— bass, bluefish, caviar, oysters.

Cramps—Lower Back Pain

These symptoms occur once menstruation begins. Many women experience menstrual cramps, as well as pain in the lower back and inner thighs. In more severe cases, a woman may experience diarrhea, nausea, vomiting, and heavy bleeding.

Menstrual cramping is caused by a predominance of Series II prostaglandins (described in more detail in the section "Meat and Poultry," on page 7). Prostaglandins are hormonelike substances produced in the uterus; the Series II prostaglandins promote contraction of the blood vessels within the uterus and the surrounding muscles. Fluid and sodium retention can also contribute to severe cramping.

Food choices: seafood, shellfish, legumes and whole grains, plus nondairy milk-like products such as nut and soy milks—avoid red meat and dairy-rich foods—fresh vegetables and fruits for fiber; unprocessed foods naturally low in salt; maple syrup rather than refined sugar.

Nutrients: magnesium—lima beans, Great Northern beans, spinach, beet greens, figs, cashews, buckwheat, shrimp; calcium—figs, papayas, canned sardines with bones, turnip greens, kidney beans, cornmeal.

Foods that Cause PMS and Those that Can Come to Your Rescue

Are you relying on fast food for many of your meals? Do you snack on potato chips or jelly beans? How often do you cook a wholesome meal at home? The basic rule of healthy eating is to eat food of the highest quality—fresh, natural, unprocessed, unrefined, and free of chemicals such as preservatives, artificial flavors, and artificial colors. Thousands of food products on the market don't meet these standards, and it takes a watchful shopper to avoid them.

The flavor of whole food is easy to like, but even more important, as you begin to eat this way, you'll also start feeling better and have fewer menstrual problems. When food is refined, a majority of vitamins, minerals, phytohormones, and other nutrients are destroyed before the food ever reaches your shopping cart. However, *whole food is your ally.*

Grains and Baked Goods

To lessen and eliminate symptoms of PMS, unrefined grains are key. When you shop, look for the word "whole." Unrefined "whole" grains provide vitamins and minerals for general good health and prevent problems associated with PMS. Fortunately, in the last few years whole-grain products have started to become widely available. Look in supermarkets and natural-food stores for such items as **whole-grain English muffins, croissants, pasta,** and hot and cold **breakfast cereals,** as well as a great variety of **whole-grain breads.** You will find these items made with whole grains such as **brown rice, whole wheat, rye, barley, oats,** etc.

When grain is refined, the bran and germ are removed, and only the central portion of the grain is retained. This is not like removing the shell from a nut, throwing away an inedible outside casing and saving a nutritious core. Bran contains fiber and many B vitamins, and the germ is full of healthy oils, vitamin E, and other nutrients, while the core of the grain, in fact, is mostly starch. The fiber in bran helps sweep excess estrogen from the intestines, thereby helping balance hormone levels. Similarly, the B vitamins support the liver in breaking down excess estrogen.

Become a label reader. What you don't want is "white flour," or "unbromated, unbleached wheat flour." You'll also see the word "enriched" on breads, which indicates that only some of the vitamins and minerals removed in processing have been added back into the refined flour. (For specific amounts of vitamins and minerals in refined and whole flour, please refer to the Appendix.)

Vegetables and Salads

Keep fresh vegetables and salad greens on hand; packaged salad, bottled beans, or frozen peas can work when you are pressed for time. Come home with a bag full of seasonal vegetables and greens, and we promise your body will thank you. Vegetables contain fiber, which is a must for the PMS diet because it helps regulate estrogen levels and prevent menstrual anxiety, irritability, and mood swings. Shop for lettuce greens such as **romaine, butter lettuce,** and **arugula,** plus **asparagus, spinach, mushrooms, potatoes, sweet potatoes,** and **dark leafy greens,** such as **kale, collards,** and **turnip greens.** In addition, try sea vegetables—yes, seaweed. **Nori** and **kelp (kombu)** contain B vitamins, vitamin E, copper, iron, magnesium, and zinc, all nutrients that promote a healthy monthly cycle. Add a little to a soup or stew, as in Terrine of Blazin' Adzuki Beans and Squash (see page 73). A small amount won't change the flavor of a dish, but it will boost its nutrition.

Meat and Poultry

Many women feel their PMS symptoms intensify after they consume red meat. Beef contains relatively high amounts of arachidonic acid, an essential fatty acid that is a normal constituent of cell membranes. Arachidonic acid converts to Series II prostaglandins, hormonelike compounds that trigger menstrual cramps, inflammation, abdominal bloating, breast tenderness, increased thirst, a craving for salty foods, and even migraines! These effects are normally counterbalanced by the Series I and

Series III prostaglandins. Oils found in vegetables, fish, seeds, and nuts convert to these prostaglandins.

Eating red meat regularly can also affect hormonal balance because of its high fat content. An excess of fat taxes the liver, which is the organ that helps regulate hormone levels, and animal fats also promote reabsorption of estrogens as they pass through the intestine for excretion.

If you do have a craving for meat, better alternatives are **lamb** and **pork.** While most cuts of these meats have a high fat content, lamb and pork do contain less arachidonic acid. However, poultry, whether **chicken** or **turkey,** is the best choice of all. Chicken contains only half the arachidonic acid of beef, and both chicken and turkey have far less fat than other meats. Therefore, as you begin the dietary changes we recommend, it is important to monitor how you feel to find which foods work best for you. You may even feel you can tolerate beef once in a while. Choose a lean cut and have a small portion, 3 to 4 ounces, equivalent to a hamburger patty the size of the palm of your hand.

Try to cook with naturally raised meat and poultry. Animals are often given synthetic estrogens to stimulate their growth. When you consume some of the supplemental hormones, you can throw off your body's own hormonal balance even more.

Dairy Foods

Like meat, dairy products such as milk and cheese are high in fat and consuming these foods may also lead to the production of symptom-causing Series II prostaglandins. Milk products can cause fluid retention and bloating, and are associated with a deficiency of dopamine, a hormone which normally promotes the excretion of fluids. Many cheeses, such as cottage cheese and blue cheese, are also often very high in sodium, which induces fluid retention. In addition, the high amount of calcium in these foods interferes with magnesium absorption, a mineral intimately involved in menstrual health. Women with a high intake of dairy foods characteristically have PMS-related nervous tension, mood swings, irritability, anxiety, and menstrual cramps. Even women consuming only low-fat dairy foods report many of these symptoms.

Nondairy milk and cheese products may be found on the market. If you crave something "creamy," you might try some of the new substitute milks made from almonds, rice, oats, and soy. Or eliminate dairy foods from your diet until your PMS symptoms abate, and then, from time to time, have some of the very best organic cheese you can find—**ricotta, fresh mozzarella, pecorino Romano,** or perhaps a round of **chèvre** rolled in *herbes de Provence*! Small amounts of top-quality cheese appear in some recipes; others feature plain **yogurt** with living cultures as an ingredient. The friendly bacteria aid digestion, and yogurt is also a good source of vitamin B12 for healthy nerves.

Fresh and Dried Fruit

Fruit contains various nutrients, each with its special benefits. **Berries** and **citrus** are high in flavonoids, which have a chemical activity similar to estrogen, while **figs, papaya, mangoes,** and **peaches** provide PMS nutrients such as the B-complex vitamins and magnesium. It is easy to eat a variety of fruit just by changing the assortment season by season. In addition, keep on hand a supply of minimally processed **dried fruits**—the unsulphured kind.

Fruit eases menstrual symptoms in several ways. Compared with refined sugar, the sugar in fruit causes only a relatively small rise in blood sugar because of the way your body stores sugar from fruit and then slowly converts it to energy. Plus the fiber contained in fruit slows its digestion and absorption, and as a result, you are less likely to feel irritable and fatigued.

Fish and Shellfish

Fish contain healthy oils, the omega-3 essential fatty acids that help prevent menstrual discomfort such as cramping. The fish with the highest content are native to cold waters, such as **salmon, tuna, mackerel, sardines,** and **herring.** Shellfish like **shrimp, crab,** and **oysters** are great sources of minerals good for keeping PMS at bay. Buy only the freshest, sweetest-smelling fish, preferably from a store that specializes in selling seafood. Another acceptable option is flash-frozen fish. Keep canned tuna and salmon on hand for healthy quick meals.

Beans and Peas

To reduce the amount of meat and dairy foods in your diet and still provide yourself with sufficient protein, include more beans and peas in your meals. These plant foods, known collectively as legumes, are a low-fat source of high-quality protein when served with whole grains. When you replace red meat with a savory bean stew, you avoid triggering PMS symptoms and initiate body chemistry that leads to a far less troublesome monthly cycle. Legumes, such as **lima beans,** which are high in magnesium, provide extra amounts of certain vitamins and minerals that help prevent PMS symptoms.

There are a wide range of dried beans and peas available in most supermarkets. Experiment with some of the bean recipes, and legumes will soon become a delicious staple in your kitchen. Also remember to order **beans** and **lentils** when you dine out on Mexican and Indian food. (You need not avoid beans if they are a problem food for you because of gas. On page 70, we tell you how to prepare and cook beans to make them more digestible.)

Nuts and Seeds

Nuts and seeds are fine foods for everyday snacking. They are great sources of healthy fats and nutrients. (See nutrient chart on page 235.) The only exception is for those who have menstrually related skin problems. Eating quantities of nuts and seeds during the ten or twelve days before your menses can aggravate complexion problems. However, after menstruation commences, during the first half of your cycle, you can enjoy a variety of nuts and seeds. **Walnuts** in particular are recommended, as they contain the omega-3 essential fatty acids. (See "Fats and Oils," page 11.)

The healthiest kinds of nuts and seeds are raw and unroasted. The oils in these nuts are of high quality and have not been altered by heat. Salted nuts or those coated with sugar can increase water retention and premenstrual weight gain. You'll find **almonds, pumpkinseeds,** and **sunflower seeds** in many of the recipes as flavor accents.

Hot and Cold Beverages

Beverages on the PMS menu include **caffeine-free herbal tea, bottled mineral waters,** and **purified water** from your home tap, fitted with a filtering device. **Fruit** and **vegetable juices** are also good choices, especially freshly made with an electric juicer-extractor. Second best are the wonderful array of unsweetened, natural juices and juice combinations now on the market. But please read labels and avoid juice drinks that include refined sugars such as high-fructose corn syrup, a form of processed sugar.

Off the PMS menu are beverages that contain caffeine, including coffee, tea, chocolate drinks, and caffeinated colas. Caffeine has a powerful effect on the nervous system and can trigger nervousness and irritability, as well as fatigue. Normally, when stress activates the adrenals, these glands stimulate the body to produce energy. When the body begins to tire, the adrenals then signal the body to slow down. It's no news to any devoted coffee drinker that caffeine overrides this protective shutdown mechanism. However, using caffeine in this way for energy can eventually result in exhaustion, a condition which can only worsen symptoms of PMS. Even decaffeinated coffee and tea are not recommended for a PMS diet. Coffee and tea, with or without caffeine, are also diuretics, increasing urination and excretion of the vitamins and minerals carried in the urine. Decaffeinated colas contain high quantities of refined sugar, which gives us a quick rush of energy and then a drop as blood sugar rises and dips. These highs and lows of blood sugar also can exaggerate emotional symptoms of PMS. (For more on sugar, see "Sugars and Sweeteners," page 11.)

Fats and Oils

Of all the components of the diet, fat is the most misunderstood. Certain fats are critical for many body functions, including normal brain activity and breathing, and play a role in hormone balance. Such useful substances are not foods to be feared! Fats and oils appear in these recipes, about 25 to 30 percent of calories on average, to enhance flavor and satisfy appetite. However, the one guideline you do need to follow is to *eat only quality fats and oils*.

For general good health, and especially for PMS, choose those fats and oils that do not contain *trans* fatty acids, molecules generated when fat is exposed to high temperatures during processing or cooking. A *trans* fatty acid is a misshapen, unnatural molecule that performs poorly when taken up by our cells. The end result is that tissues and eventually organs may malfunction, and heart disease and perhaps even cancer can develop. In terms of PMS, *trans* fatty acids block the production of Series I prostaglandins that ease menstrual symptoms such as fluid retention, irritability, depression, low blood sugar, and carbohydrate cravings. These altered fats are found in margarine, in all food products that include the word "hydrogenated" in the ingredients list, and in all fried foods.

You also need to make sure you are consuming sufficient quantities of essential fatty acids (EFA's), oils found in vegetables, seeds, and fish. The oils (omega-3 EFA's) found in **fish, flaxseeds,** and **walnuts** are converted to beneficial prostaglandins that are particularly effective in preventing menstrual cramping.

The fats and oils that meet these standards are **butter, extra-virgin olive oil,** and **flaxseed oil.** We avoid margarine and refined vegetable oil. (For a complete description of fats and oils, please refer to the Appendix.)

Sugars and Sweeteners

Cross off refined white sugar from your shopping list! Instead, stock up on natural sweeteners such as pure **maple syrup** (not "pancake" syrup, which is made of corn syrup) and **raw honey.** The manufacturing process that refines white sugar removes essential vitamins and minerals and leaves only the calories! Furthermore, the body uses B vitamins and magnesium to metabolize sugar and produce energy, and robs its reserves of these nutrients to do this. Having sufficient levels of B vitamins and magnesium is necessary for maintaining a symptom-free monthly cycle. Refined sugar also promotes the excretion of magnesium in the urine.

The dramatic highs and lows of blood sugar induced by an excess of refined sugar can trigger PMS symptoms such as mood swings, anxiety, irritability, and heart palpitations. Low blood sugar can lead to PMS depression and bouts of crying, as well as mental confusion and forgetfulness. Refined sugars can even promote fluid retention, bloating, breast tenderness, and swollen ankles.

Eating sugary foods increases the amount of serotonin the brain produces, a substance that steadies and elevates mood. But the same effect can be achieved by eating such healthful complex carbohydrates as **brown rice, barley, millet,** and root vegetables such as **sweet potatoes, carrots, white potatoes,** and **parsnips.** Do yourself a favor and on a monthly calendar, jot down a reminder to eat the healthy carbohydrates for those five to ten days just before you expect to have your period. You'll be more likely to avoid a brownie binge!

Salt and Seasonings

The PMS diet is low salt. The intake of common table salt, or sodium chloride, causes the body to retain fluids. As water accumulates in tissues, swollen ankles and abdominal bloating result. To prevent such symptoms, lower salt intake during the seven to ten days before menses begins, and switch from sodium chloride to sea salt. Women we have counseled about PMS report that when they use sea salt they are less likely to retain fluid.

There are also other ways to heighten flavor besides relying on salt alone. Try a squeeze of **lemon** on asparagus, **garlic** and **pepper** in the mashed potatoes, or a splash of **extra-virgin olive oil** and **fresh herbs** in your bean soup. In addition, herbal sea salt is a quick and easy way to add a more complex flavor accent that blends well with most dishes.

Vitamins and Minerals for PMS—the Pick of the Crop

The following gives you an overview of the vitamins and minerals recommended for a PMS-free diet, which foods contain especially high amounts of the nutrients, and which PMS symptoms they treat. As you begin to cook, you'll notice these foods again and again as the primary ingredients. Gradually, you will familiarize yourself with the specific nutrients that treat your particular symptoms.

Vitamin A

That beautiful display of winter squash—**butternut, acorn, Hubbard**—with their golden-orange interiors; a mound of **carrots** with their lacy tops; as well as **mangos, papaya, cantaloupe,** and **sweet potatoes** are all great sources of vitamin A. The form of vitamin A in plants is beta-carotene, a rich yellow-orange pigment, and many foods with this color are a good source. Green vegetables such as **broccoli, spinach,** and **bok choy** also contain beta-carotene. Vitamin A itself is in animal foods such as **eggs, butter,** and **calves' liver** (buy only organic).

Vitamin A on the Menu
- Cathy's Easy Fresh-fruit Salad (see page 217)
- Skillet-roasted Sweet Potatoes, Carrots, and Parsnips with Rosemary (see page 125)

> *Vitamin A: reduces fluid retention, abdominal bloating, and swollen breasts; helps prevent fatigue and lessens heavy menstrual flow.*

B-complex Vitamins

The B-complex vitamins include thiamin (B1), riboflavin (B2), niacin (B3), pantothenic acid (B5), pyridoxine (B6), cobalamin (B12), pangamic acid (B15), biotin, choline, folic acid, inositol, and para-aminobenzoic acid (PABA). You'll find these vitamins in **whole grains, organ meats, blackstrap molasses,** and **dark leafy greens** such as **kale.** Many of the B vitamins are also found in **eggs, beans,** and **dairy products** such as **yogurt.**

Vitamin B-complex on the Menu
- Caribbean Twice-cooked Pinto Beans with Plantains (see page 76)
- Fresh Tuna Salad Sandwiches (see page 191)

> *Vitamin B: stabilizes PMS mood swings, manages stress and helps to prevent irritability and fatigue; and reduces heavy menstrual bleeding.*

Vitamin B6

If you are shopping for vitamin B6, head for the meat and poultry section. **Beef, pork,** and **poultry,** including **chicken, turkey, duck, quail,** and **pheasant,** all contain plentiful vitamin B6.

Another good source are **whole grains** such as **brown rice** and **whole wheat.** Whole-wheat flour has over six times more vitamin B6 than white enriched wheat flour. And don't forget these B6 foods—**beans, broccoli, bananas,** and **blackstrap molasses.**

Vitamin B6 on the Menu
- Lima Beans, Corn, and Green Bean Succotash (see page 79)
- Bulgur Pilaf with Cremini Mushrooms and Roasted Sunflower Seeds (see page 91)

> *Vitamin B6: helps to prevent mood swings, irritability, depression, abdominal bloating; counteracts cravings for sugar and reduces fatigue. Needed for the metabolism of estrogen.*

Choline and Inositol

When you add **whole grains, citrus fruits, unsulphured molasses, fish, tofu,** and **nuts** to your shopping list, you'll come home with foods that contain these two nutrients, which are part of the vitamin B-complex. There's lots of choline in **egg yolks,** one of the many good reasons not to buy egg substitutes made only from egg whites.

Choline and Inositol on the Menu
- Vegetable Paella Primer (see page 87)
- Texan Two-step Chili (see page 72)

> *Choline and Inositol: relieves irritability, mood swings, and fluid retention. Inositol has a sedating effect on the central nervous system, lessening menstrual anxiety.*

Vitamin C

Everyone knows that **citrus** fruit contains vitamin C, but were you aware that many other fruits and vegetables are equally good sources? One cup of any of the following contains as much vitamin C as one orange: **strawberries, papaya, broccoli, cauliflower,** and **sweet red** and **green peppers.**

Vitamin C on the Menu
- Ukrainian Cabbage and Potatoes with Fresh Herbs (see page 120)
- Sesame Lemon Snaps with Almonds (see page 209)

> *Vitamin C: reduces heavy menstrual bleeding and helps combat stress that can tax the nervous system and increase irritability; increases iron absorption to prevent anemia.*

Flavonoids

Flavonoids are a group of water-soluble vitamins that behave like estrogens and have a low-potency hormonal effect. Go for the gold and invest in some **apricots, cherries, plums,** and luxurious **blackberries,** as well as other **berries** of the season, to put flavonoids in your shopping cart. Flavonoids are also plentiful in all **citrus** and in **buckwheat,** sold packaged as the grain **kasha,** or as noodles called **soba.** You'll find these in the rice and pasta aisles in the natural-food store.

Flavonoids on the Menu
- Roasted Chicken with Kasha and Wild Mushroom Stuffing (see page 150)
- Fresh Blueberry Marzipan Tart with Orange Glaze (see page 219)

> *Flavonoids: lessens heavy menstrual bleeding and cramping and prevents fluid retention, headaches, and mood swings.*

Vitamin E

Vitamin E is the woman's vitamin, having a significant effect on the hormone system. Buy unprocessed ingredients such as **whole grains** and **eggs** from free-range chickens. If you don't find these items in your regular supermarket, here's a great reason to explore your neighborhood for a natural-food store that will tend to carry more vitamin E–rich products. **Cucumber, kale, fresh peas,** and **nuts** such as **hazelnuts** and **almonds** are also good sources.

Vitamin E on the Menu
- Creamy Hungarian Asparagus Soup (see page 28)
- Clam and Shrimp Bouillabaisse (see page 144)

> *Vitamin E: relieves breast tenderness, food cravings related to PMS, and emotional symptoms such as depression and anxiety.*

Calcium

There are calcium foods everywhere in the store, not just in the dairy section. We recommend you stock up on plain **yogurt** (there's about 300 mg of calcium per cup), but you'll also find calcium in **broccoli, spinach,** the **leafy tops of beets** and

turnips, cabbage, and even **okra.** At the fish counter there is calcium in the fresh **shrimp** and **oysters.** As a convenient backup food for lunch, a good choice is fish that is canned with bones intact, such as **salmon, sardines,** and **mackerel.**

Calcium on the Menu
- Louisiana Greens Gumbo (see page 30)
- Yogurt Herb Dressing (see page 62)

Calcium: lessens painful cramps, generalized aches and pains, psychological symptoms, food cravings, and fluid retention as well as promoting restful sleep. Calcium is a good menu choice during the two weeks of the cycle before menstruation, when blood levels of calcium may decline.

Magnesium

You can always spot the magnesium in the produce section of the market—the greener the fruit or vegetable, the more magnesium it contains. So reach for those bunches of **kale, collards,** and **turnip greens! Potatoes, black-eyed peas, avocados, figs,** and especially **lima beans** are also good sources. And you'll bring home magnesium foods when you put **fish,** all kinds of **nuts,** and **pumpkinseeds** in your shopping cart. Women with PMS typically have low magnesium reserves.

Magnesium on the Menu
- Black Bean Timbales with Pumpkinseeds (see page 75)
- Complete Meal Bulgur Salad (see page 57)

Magnesium: reduces irritability and mood swings. Maintains normal levels of dopamine, a neurotransmitter in the brain that helps regulate emotions. Facilitates sugar metabolism and curbs sugar cravings, lessens cramps, and prevents inflammation associated with breast tenderness.

Iron

Both plant foods and meats contain iron, but the kind in animal protein is better absorbed. To give your blood a quick, hefty boost, if you find you can tolerate red meat, buy some **organic liver** or **fish.** Plant foods that are good sources of iron include **parsley, leeks, peas, artichokes, raisins,** and **peaches.**

Iron on the Menu
- French Bistro Entrecôte (see page 156)
- Silky Peach Custard with Pistachios and Cardamom Swirl (see page 215)

Iron: replenishes iron in the blood lost because of heavy menstrual bleeding, restoring energy and stamina.

Zinc

Oysters are so high in this mineral that eating an oyster is equivalent to taking a zinc supplement. There's also zinc in **crab,** but not the imitation kind, surimi, made from white fish. Order these when you are dining out, and if you are doing the cooking, buy some **fresh corn, mushrooms,** or **lima beans** to put some zinc on your plate. **Pumpkinseeds, sunflower seeds,** and **pecans** also make good zinc snacks.

Zinc on the Menu
- Curried Chicken and Vegetable Stir-fry (see page 152)
- Phyto Rice and Quinoa Salad (see page 55)

Zinc: reduces irritability and depression. When zinc is deficient and copper in excess, this can lead to moodiness. Facilitates the use of vitamin B6 and the EFA's.

Take Time to Nurture Yourself and Enjoy the Results

Give yourself the gift of eating peacefully at least once a day. Being in a relaxed state eases your body's digestion and improves the absorption of nutrients, quelling PMS symptoms. Your busy schedule may require grabbing some meals on the run, but you can create a little oasis here and there. If you work in a congested urban setting, seek out a quiet corner to eat your lunch. At home, put a flower on the table and light a candle. Do not eat on a dining table cluttered with work papers, and resist the temptation of eating at your desk or while working at the computer.

You may also want to try more focused stress reduction. Some women take an early morning walk or a stroll after dinner, practice yoga, meditation, or focused breathing, and have a massage once a week. Such self-care can ease menstrual symptoms such as cramps and irritability.

A woman who takes the time to eat the right foods (and eliminate harmful ones) can look forward to long-term health. Whether you alter your diet all at once, or make changes step by step, you will find a pace that is right for you. Enjoy immediate benefits from certain changes like going off caffeine. Some women also find that their severe menstrual cramps cease in just a month or two after they've stopped eating red meat. Allow your process six to twelve cycles to evolve, as you learn to shop for new ingredients and use the recipes in this book.

It's a good idea to keep mental notes of how you feel from month to month, even jotting these down on your calendar. As symptoms diminish, you'll find it easier to stick with your new dietary patterns, and if a symptom persists, you'll know to be more aggressive in trying to eliminate it.

It's interesting—though it might sound strange at first—to learn to dialogue with your body. When you have a craving for a certain food, such as chocolate cake, ask yourself whether you really want the fat in the cake, the sugar, the caffeine in the chocolate, or the bitter taste. Your body may even be craving the chocolate's magnesium. Identifying what it is really hungry for can help you figure out the most healthful way to give this to yourself. It also pays to notice how you feel after eating a particular food. Monitor your PMS symptoms, such as irritability and headaches, for the next day or two to notice if symptoms worsen. We acknowledge that sometimes the only thing that will fix a chocolate-cake craving is chocolate cake, but when it comes to the day-to-day cravings, it's a good idea to think in terms of substitutions. For rich and bitter flavors, enjoy toasted and grilled foods and dark greens such as kale. For coffee, substitute grain beverages. Baked beans and pumpkinseeds will supply magnesium, and crunching on popcorn can give an energy boost. As you eat the way we recommend, we guarantee you'll soon reach a new level of health and well-being throughout the month.

Cooking that Cures

Now that you have some familiarity with how food affects your menstrual cycle, it's your turn to use this information and have it work for you. If you rarely cook, we invite you into the kitchen. Review the symptoms, food groups, and nutrient sections of this introduction, then take a look at "PMS Foods to the Rescue!" in the Appendix (see page 247) and write a shopping list of foods that cater to your monthly needs. Pay a visit to a farmer's market for the freshest produce of the season or explore the many intriguing new products in your local natural-food store.

You might find that you use this book first to address PMS, and then notice that family and friends enjoy and benefit from the meals as well.

Now, it's time to put on your apron!

All in One Pot

Soups

South Indian Curry Soup with Greens   23

Velvet Black Bean Soup with Corn Relish   24

Chunky Vegetable Minestrone with Cannellini Beans   26

Mushroom Bouquet Soup with Wild Rice   27

Creamy Hungarian Asparagus Soup   28

Louisiana Greens Gumbo   30

Yellow Split-Pea Soup with Buttercup Squash Chunks   32

Stocks

Vegetable Stock au Bouquet Garni   33

Light Fish Stock   35

Beef Bone or Poultry Stock   36

Stews

Cajun Red Lentil and Corn Stew   37

Three-Bean Vegetarian Cassoulet   39

Four-Onion and Red-Bean Vegetable Tagine   41

Multi-Potato Stew with Beef and Lamb Cubes   42

Sweet Potato and Turnip Stew with Chicken Strips   44

Creating a Balanced Meal with Soups

Vegetarian meal planning is simple when you know and understand the basics. Beans combined with a whole grain provides quality protein equivalent to red meat. For the highest quality plant protein, the basic rule of thumb is to consume grains and beans in a proportion of 1½ to 2 parts whole grains to 1 part beans, or ¾ to 1 cup cooked grain to ½ cup cooked beans. If you mix grains with seeds or nuts to form a complete protein, add 1 cup cooked grain to 2 tablespoons seeds or nuts. To benefit from such combinations, you don't necessarily have to eat the grains and beans at the same meal, just in the same day. Even if you're not vegetarian, it's a good idea to have a whole grain with your protein food to add vitamins and fiber to your diet, as well as beans on a daily basis for their minerals and soluble fiber.

- Bean soup or stew as the center of the meal, plus a grain product such as a slice of whole wheat bread, cooked brown rice, or a side of polenta (cornmeal mush).
- To a light vegetable soup, add some whole-grain pita wedges topped with nut butter or bean spread.
- A rich and hearty soup like a gumbo or a chowder plus a side salad.
- Any leftover stew turns into a soup, just by adding water or homemade stock and a little additional seasoning—a perfect way to finish leftovers.

Sides for Soup

You can serve many whole-grain items with soup. Look for good-quality sliced breads, pitas, croissants, English muffins, baguettes, bread sticks, corn or whole wheat tortillas. There are also simple preparations that you can add to toasted breads to make *bruschetta*.

To prepare bruschetta, lightly toast sliced bread, baguettes, or pita, and top with any of the following. After the topping has been added, the bruschetta can be baked in a toaster oven for several minutes. Serve these alongside a bowl of homemade soup and you'll have family and friends knocking at your door!

- Rub the toast with peeled raw garlic and drizzle with extra-virgin olive oil; sprinkle with basil and a pinch of herbal sea salt.
- Spread almond butter on the toast and top with avocado slices and a few drops of lemon juice.
- Place a thin slice of French Lentil and Walnut Pâté (see page 194) on the toast and top with a slice of fresh tomato.
- Spread the toast with tahini, apple butter, and a few grains of sea salt.

What to Do with Leftover Cooked Beans

Soup: Use leftover cooked beans to make soup by adding purified water or homemade stock, season to taste, and add any one or a combination of the following suggestions:

1. Add your favorite chopped vegetables.
2. Puree the beans and liquid to give a creamy texture.
3. Puree part of the soup (one-quarter to one-half) to give a thicker consistency.
4. Add pasta or a grain (already cooked is the fastest) to create a complete protein.
5. Add your favorite spice mixture, such as curry or chili powder, garam masala, or any bottled herb mixtures, such as Italian, Asian, or Provençal combinations.

Twice-cooked beans: Heat a little extra-virgin olive oil or butter in a frying pan and add chopped onion and garlic, spices, leftover cooked beans, and some bean liquid, stock, or water. Mash the beans with the back of a wooden spoon and cook uncovered, until the beans have almost fallen apart, about 20 minutes. Stir occasionally and add additional liquid if the mixture begins to dry out. **Spice suggestions:** Whether you are making soup or twice-cooked beans, these spices will help flavor the dish—curry powder, chili powder, basil and oregano, or rosemary.

Bean Soup Soaking and Cooking Chart

A simple rule of thumb for cooking beans is 1 cup dried beans makes 2 to 2½ cups of soaked or cooked beans (see pages 69–71 for complete instructions). In the recipes, we will specify 1 cup of dried beans, and whatever volume the beans become after soaking, it's all right to use them all.

Bean name	Soak	Soup cooking time*
Adzuki beans	no	1 to 1½ hours
Adzuki beans	yes	45 minutes
Black beans	yes	50 to 60 minutes
Black-eyed peas	yes	45 minutes
Cannellini beans	yes	60 minutes
Chickpeas	yes	1 to 1½ hours
Great Northern beans	yes	50 to 60 minutes
Kidney beans	yes	60 minutes

*The specifications are for 1 cup of dried beans.

Bean name	Soak	Soup cooking time*
Lentils, green	no	45 minutes
Navy beans	yes	50 minutes
Pinto beans	yes	55 minutes
Red lentils	no	20 minutes
Split peas	no	1½ hours

 # South Indian Curry Soup with Greens

Yield: 6 servings   100% vegetarian

This flavorful soup is a simple way to incorporate a rich nutrient base of vitamins and minerals with lots of fiber.

PMS Benefits: Magnesium assists the body in calcium and potassium absorption, stabilizes moods, increases energy, and decreases PMS sugar cravings and cramps. The leafy greens featured in this recipe contain a good amount of magnesium.

2 **cups red lentils, sorted and washed (see Note)**
6 **cups purified water or homemade salt-free vegetable stock**
2 **tablespoons curry powder**
1 **bay leaf**
2 **stalks celery, chopped**
1 **onion, chopped**
1 **carrot, ends trimmed, chopped**
2 **cloves garlic, minced**
1 **tablespoon ghee (see page 227) or unsalted butter, preferably organic**
1 **teaspoon herbal sea salt**
¼ **teaspoon ground pepper**
   Approximately 4 cups chopped greens, such as spinach, chard,
      watercress, arugula, or bok choy

1. In a large soup pot, bring the red lentils, water or stock, curry powder, and bay leaf to a boil. Cover, reduce flame, and simmer for 10 minutes.

2. Add the celery, onion, carrot, and garlic to the soup and stir well. Continue cooking until the lentils fall apart, about another 15 minutes.

3. Add the ghee or butter, herbal sea salt, and pepper and stir. Add the greens just before serving. They will wilt quickly in the hot soup but maintain their green color.

(South Indian Curry Soup with Greens—Continued)

Taste and add more herbal sea salt, if desired. Serve with a bottle of hot sauce on the side, for those who dare!

Cooking Tip: Curry is usually cooked before adding it to a dish to blend in the flavors. To avoid this step, add the curry with the lentils at the beginning of the cooking time. This will prevent the oil from cooking twice (during the toasting and while the soup is cooking), avoid the possibility of the spices burning, and give you one less utensil to clean!

Note: Instead of the red lentils, you can substitute soaked dried beans such as Great Northern, pinto, or chickpeas.

Nutritional Stars: Magnesium, folic acid, B-complex vitamins

 # Velvet Black Bean Soup with Corn Relish

Yield: 6 servings   100% vegetarian

A very tasty wake-up dish that can turn dinner into a party!

PMS Benefits: Niacin (vitamin B3) maintains healthy-looking skin and healthy nerves. Iron helps the body to build blood and counteract anemia caused by heavy menstrual flow. Black beans are a good source of both nutrients.

Before you begin, soak 1 cup sorted and washed dried black beans in a bowl with 5 cups of purified water for 6 hours or overnight.

The soup:

    2 cups soaked black beans (from 1 cup dried beans)
    5 cups purified water or homemade salt-free vegetable stock
    1 strip kombu seaweed or bay leaf
    2 cloves garlic, minced
    1 potato, peeled and cut into chunks
    1 ripe beefsteak tomato or 2 plum tomatoes, cores removed, diced
    1 onion, chopped
    1 carrot, ends trimmed, chopped
    2 to 3 tablespoons extra-virgin olive oil or unsalted butter, preferably
        organic
    1 teaspoon herbal sea salt
    ¼ teaspoon ground pepper

The relish:

2 ears fresh corn, husked and kernels removed from the cob
½ cup purified water
1 red onion, chopped fine
2 cloves garlic, minced
2 tablespoons cider vinegar
2 to 3 sprigs fresh cilantro (coriander), washed, thick stems removed,
    chopped
1 teaspoon hot sauce, if desired
½ teaspoon herbal sea salt
    Ground pepper

The soup:

1. With your hands or a slotted spoon, remove the beans from the soaking water and put them into a large soup pot with the water or stock and kombu or bay leaf. Bring to a boil, reduce flame, and simmer with the lid slightly uncovered, for 30 minutes.

2. Add the garlic, potato, tomato, onion, and carrot. Return to a boil, lower flame, and continue to simmer covered until the beans and potato are tender, another 15 to 20 minutes. Meanwhile, prepare the relish.

3. In a blender or food processor, puree the soup in small batches, pouring each blenderful into another pot or bowl, until the entire soup is smooth. Puree the kombu with the beans (or discard the bay leaf). Be careful when blending hot soup. (After covering the blender or processor with the container's lid, place a kitchen towel over the top of the container to catch any hot liquid that may spray out and burn you.)

4. Add the oil, herbal sea salt, and pepper. If a thinner consistency is desired, stir additional water or stock into the pureed soup (or add the corn stock after making the relish). Check for seasoning, and add salt and pepper to taste, if desired.

5. Ladle into bowls and top with 1 or 2 tablespoons Corn Relish; serve with extra hot sauce on the side.

The relish:

1. In a small saucepan, put the corn kernels and the water. Bring to a boil covered, reduce flame, and simmer until softened, 3 or 4 minutes. Turn off the flame and add the onion and garlic (this will take a little of the bite out, or if you prefer, add them raw after draining the corn), and leave covered for about 5 minutes.

2. Place a colander or sieve in a bowl and pour the corn mixture into it. Drain well and put in a medium bowl with the vinegar, cilantro, hot sauce, herbal sea salt, and a few grinds or shakes of pepper. Stir and set aside. Add the drained corn stock to the pureed soup, if desired.

(Velvet Black Bean Soup with Corn Relish—Continued)
Cooking Tip: Do not add salt to beans until they are fully cooked or they will stay hard, even after the recommended cooking period.
Nutritional Stars: Niacin, folic acid, iron

 # Chunky Vegetable Minestrone with Cannellini Beans

Yield: 6 servings   100% vegetarian

Rich with colors, textures, and nutrients, this soup is a full meal. Serve it with a green salad and some whole-grain bread sticks for a very satisfying lunch or light dinner.

PMS Benefits: Magnesium is needed to optimize calcium absorption in the body. If you have PMS cramps, sugar cravings, or mood swings, shop for some cannellini beans and spinach, which contain both of these minerals.

Before you begin, soak 1 cup sorted and washed dried cannellini beans in a bowl with 5 cups of purified water for 6 hours or overnight.

> **2 cups soaked cannellini beans (from 1 cup dried beans)**
> **6 cups purified water or homemade salt-free vegetable stock**
> **1 bay leaf**
> **2 tomatoes, cores removed, chopped**
> **2 stalks celery, diced**
> **2 cloves garlic, minced**
> **1 onion, diced**
> **1 carrot, ends trimmed, diced**
> **1 green bell pepper, seeded and diced**
> **1 red bell pepper, seeded and diced**
> **1 turnip or black radish, cut into chunks**
> **6 to 8 button mushrooms, cut in half**
> **1 teaspoon dried basil or marjoram**
> **½ teaspoon dried thyme**
> **1 bunch spinach, ends trimmed, washed, and chopped coarsely**
> **1 teaspoon herbal sea salt**
> **¼ teaspoon ground pepper**

1. With your hands or a slotted spoon, remove the beans from the soaking water and put them in a large soup pot with the fresh water or stock and bay leaf. Bring to a boil on a high flame, reduce flame, and simmer with the lid partly uncovered, about 30 minutes.

2. Add the tomatoes, celery, garlic, onion, carrot, green and red peppers, turnip or black radish, mushroom halves, basil or marjoram, and thyme. Return to a boil, reduce flame, and cook covered until the beans and vegetables are tender, another 15 to 20 minutes. Stir occasionally.

3. Add the spinach and stir, cooking for another 2 minutes. Discard the bay leaf. Season with the herbal sea salt and pepper, and stir well. (This soup can be partially blended, if desired. See Cooking Tip.) Ladle the soup into bowls and enjoy.

Cooking Tip: For a creamier soup base with some texture, puree up to one-third to one-half of the soup in small batches, returning the blended soup to the pot. Stir well.

Nutritional Stars: B-complex vitamins, vitamin C, folic acid, calcium, magnesium

 ## Mushroom Bouquet Soup with Wild Rice

Yield: 4 to 6 servings　　　100% vegetarian

You can use either one kind of mushroom or a mixture of several. We like to use button mushrooms, portobello, and cremini or oyster mushrooms—a total of 1 to 1½ pounds.

PMS Benefits: Pantothenic acid (vitamin B5) helps treat depression and anxiety. A deficiency of this B vitamin can lead to fatigue and headaches. The mushrooms and whole grains in this recipe contain a plentiful amount of vitamin B5.

- ½ cup wild rice, washed
- 5½ to 6 cups purified water or homemade salt-free vegetable stock
  Sea salt
- 1 portobello mushroom
- 1 8- to 10-ounce box button mushrooms, washed
- 1 onion, chopped
- 1 to 2 potatoes, peeled and cut into chunks, or ¼ cup rolled oatmeal
- 4 cloves garlic, peeled
- 1 bay leaf
- ½ teaspoon dried thyme or marjoram
- ¼ pound cremini or oyster mushrooms, washed
- 2 tablespoons unsalted butter, preferably organic, more if desired
- 1 to 2 teaspoons herbal sea salt
- 2 pinches ground white pepper
- 2 tablespoons extra-virgin olive oil

(Mushroom Bouquet Soup with Wild Rice—Continued)

1. In a small saucepan, bring the wild rice and 1½ cups purified water to a boil with a pinch of sea salt, covered. Reduce flame to a simmer and cook for 1 hour. The grains should begin to separate and curl at the ends.

2. Separate the portobello cap and stem; trim and wash. Cut both into chunks.

3. In a large soup pot, put the water or stock, portobello and button mushrooms, onion, potato or oatmeal, 2 cloves garlic, bay leaf, and thyme or marjoram. Bring to a boil, covered.

4. Remove the stems of the cremini or oyster mushrooms and set the tops aside. Add the stems to the soup. Reduce the flame and simmer until the potato is soft or the oatmeal is cooked, about 20 minutes. Turn off the flame and let sit with the cover off for 10 minutes.

5. Slice the tops of the cremini or oyster mushrooms. Mince the remaining 2 cloves garlic. Heat the butter in a skillet and add the mushrooms, garlic, 2 pinches of herbal sea salt, and a pinch of pepper. Cook on medium-low heat, covered, until the mushrooms begin to release their juice, 4 to 5 minutes. Turn off the flame and uncover the skillet.

6. Remove and discard the bay leaf. In a blender or food processor, puree the soup in small batches, pouring each blenderful into another pot or bowl until the entire soup is smooth. Be careful when blending hot soup. (After covering the blender or processor with the container's lid, place a kitchen towel over the top of the container to catch any hot liquid that may spray out and burn you.)

7. Season the soup with the olive oil, the remaining herbal sea salt, and pepper. Stir and taste the pureed soup for seasoning. (More herbal sea salt may be desired.) Add the wild rice to the mushrooms in the skillet and stir. Ladle the soup into bowls and top with 2 or 3 tablespoons of the mushroom-rice mixture. Enjoy the wonderful bouquet!

Cooking Tip: Fresh mushrooms absorb lots of water and become discolored. To avoid this, wash mushrooms quickly and use them immediately.

Nutritional Stars: B-complex vitamins, vitamin B5

 # Creamy Hungarian Asparagus Soup

Yield: 6 servings   100% vegetarian

Hungarians use paprika extensively—for soups, vegetables, meat, poultry, and fish dishes. There are at least six different kinds of this finely ground powder, ranging from the brightest red to a light rose, and the flavors span from light, sweet, and spicy to extremely sharp and hot. (PS: This soup has no cream.)

PMS Benefits: Asparagus contains high levels of folic acid, a component of the B-complex vitamins. This works to stabilize your moods and prevent irritability and fatigue. Increase your intake of fresh fruits and vegetables along with the asparagus to increase your levels of folic acid.

   1 **to 1½ pounds fresh asparagus**
   4 **cups homemade salt-free vegetable stock or purified water**
   2 **potatoes, peeled and diced, or ¼ cup rolled oatmeal**
   2 **cloves garlic, peeled**
   1 **onion, chopped**
   1 **bay leaf**
   1 **to 2 teaspoons paprika (see Cooking Tip)**
  ½ **teaspoon dried chervil or dill leaves**
   2 **tablespoons extra-virgin olive oil or unsalted butter,**
      preferably organic
   1 **teaspoon herbal sea salt**
   2 **pinches ground white pepper**

1. Break off the thick, woody asparagus ends. They will usually snap off just above the white area, which can be discarded. Remove the asparagus tips and set aside. Cut or break the asparagus stalks into thirds. In a large soup pot, bring the stock or water, asparagus stalks, potato or oatmeal, garlic, onion, bay leaf, paprika, and chervil or dill to a boil. Cook with the lid partly uncovered. Reduce heat and simmer until the vegetables are very soft, 15 to 20 minutes.

2. Remove and discard the bay leaf. Set a sieve or food mill over another pot. Using a blender or food processor, puree the soup in small batches, pouring each blenderful into the sieve. Be careful when blending hot soup. (After covering the blender or processor with the container's lid, place a kitchen towel over the top of the container to catch any hot liquid that may spray out and burn you.) Use a wooden spoon in the sieve or turn the food mill handle to separate the blended soup from the fibrous parts of the asparagus (see Note).

3. Place the pureed soup on a medium flame. Add the asparagus tips, olive oil, herbal sea salt, and pepper, and stir. Let the tips cook slightly, about 2 minutes.

4. Do not bring to a boil. Ladle the soup into bowls with two or three asparagus tips in each bowl.

Cooking Tip: Paprika is made from ground dried red peppers. The pungency of this spice depends upon the proportion of flesh to the seeds, which are hotter. If you have sweet paprika, it can be used in generous amounts, but watch out for very hot paprika—too much can ruin a dish.

(Creamy Hungarian Asparagus Soup—Continued)

Note: When preparing a creamy soup with asparagus, broccoli, celery, leeks, or other fibrous vegetables, pour them through a food mill or sieve to remove the woody and stringy parts.

Nutritional Stars: B-complex vitamins, vitamin C, folic acid

 # Louisiana Greens Gumbo

Yield: 6 to 8 servings

PMS Benefits: You can find fifteen PMS nutrients in this recipe. They include vitamins A, B1, B2, B5, B6, B12, C, E, folic acid, and flavonoids, and the minerals calcium, copper, iron, magnesium, and zinc.

- ½ **pound fresh okra, stems removed and chopped**
- 3 **tablespoons unsalted butter, preferably organic, or extra-virgin olive oil**
- ½ **teaspoon ground black pepper**
- ¼ **teaspoon ground white pepper**
- ¼ **teaspoon cayenne pepper**
- 2 **stalks celery, chopped**
- 1 **onion, chopped**
- 1 **small leek, split, washed, and chopped, both white and tender green stalks (see Cooking Tip)**
- 1 **green bell pepper, seeded and chopped**
- 6 **cups homemade salt-free fish, chicken, or vegetable stock or purified water**
- 1 **ripe tomato, core removed, chopped**
- 2 **cloves garlic, minced**
- 1 **small bunch mustard or turnip greens, washed and chopped**
- 1 **small bunch dandelion greens, collard greens, or kale, washed and chopped**
- 1 **small bunch beet greens, spinach, or chard, washed and chopped**
- ½ **teaspoon dried oregano or thyme**
- ⅛ **pound chemical-free andouille or kielbasa sausage (optional)**
- ½ **to 1 pint shucked oysters and juice**
- ½ **pound uncooked medium shrimp, peeled and deveined**
- 2 **scallions, ends trimmed, chopped or sliced**
- ½ **to 1 teaspoon sea salt**
- 2 **teaspoons lemon juice**
- ½ **teaspoon filé or sassafras powder (optional)**
  Lemon wedges
  Hot sauce

1. Set ½ cup okra aside. In a large stockpot, heat 2 tablespoons butter or oil and add all the okra except the ½ cup. Sauté on medium heat and add the black, white, and cayenne peppers. Stir frequently, cooking until the okra begins to brown, 10 to 12 minutes.

2. To the pot, add the celery, onion, leek, and green pepper, and continue sautéing for 5 more minutes. Stir occasionally, scraping the bottom of the pan with a wooden spoon.

3. Increase the heat, and add 1 cup stock. Cook uncovered for 5 minutes, stirring and scraping often.

4. Add the tomato and garlic to the pot and continue cooking, stirring frequently, another 5 minutes.

5. Add 2 more cups stock and continue cooking on a high flame, uncovered, for 5 more minutes.

6. Add the remaining 1 tablespoon butter and 3 cups stock, and return to a boil. Add the mustard or turnip greens; dandelion greens, collard greens, or kale; beet greens, spinach, or chard, with the oregano or thyme, and sausage, if using. Reduce heat and simmer covered for 45 minutes, stirring occasionally.

7. Add the remaining ½ cup okra and cook 10 minutes.

8. Place a fine mesh sieve or cheesecloth-lined colander over a bowl. Pour in the oysters and liquid. Remove the oysters from the sieve to a medium-sized bowl, as the liquid is draining. Reserve the liquid. Inspect the oysters for any remaining shell fragments.

9. Add the oysters and juice, shrimp, scallions, and salt. Stir and return to a boil, cooking for 1 or 2 more minutes, uncovered.

10. Add the lemon juice and give the gumbo one last stir.

11. Ladle the gumbo into large bowls and sprinkle each with filé or sassafras powder and serve with a lemon wedge. Offer a bottle of hot sauce, for those who like some additional heat!

Cooking Tip: To wash leeks, use a paring knife and split the white and green parts in half lengthwise, without cutting through the root. Hold the leek upside down under running water and, washing one side at a time, rub each leek leaf with your fingers, allowing the sand and soil to wash out. Once clean, cut off the roots and discard. Slice the white and tender lighter green leaves. Discard the dark green leaves or save for soup stock.

Note: To prepare this as a vegetarian soup, leave out all of the shellfish and substitute vegetable stock for the fish or chicken.

Nutritional Stars: Vitamin A, vitamin B1, vitamin B2, vitamin B5, vitamin B6, vitamin B12, vitamin C, vitamin E, folic acid, flavonoids, calcium, copper, iron, magnesium, and zinc—plus vitamin D, selenium, and omega-3 fatty acids

🍵 Yellow Split-Pea Soup with Buttercup Squash Chunks

Yield: 6 servings

Golden as the sun and rich with nutrients, this creamy soup contains soft chunks of squash, which have a luscious texture for days when you need some extra care.

PMS Benefits: The combination of zinc and vitamins A and C helps treat acne associated with PMS. Zinc is in short supply in the soil, so you need to take extra care to consume enough. You will find zinc in both the chickpea miso and the split peas used in this recipe. The golden squash supplies the vitamins C and A found in deep orange foods.

2 **cups yellow or green split peas, sorted and washed**
5 **cups purified water or homemade salt-free stock**
1 **ham hock, 4 slices bacon, or ⅛ pound pancetta, preferably chemical-free (optional)**
1 **buttercup or butternut squash**
2 **onions, chopped**
2 **to 3 cloves garlic, minced**
2 **stalks celery, ends trimmed, chopped**
1 **potato, peeled and cut into chunks**
2 **tablespoons chickpea miso**
½ **teaspoon herbal sea salt**
¼ **teaspoon ground pepper**
2 **teaspoons unsalted butter, preferably organic, or extra-virgin olive oil**
  Dill or parsley for garnishes

1. In a large soup pot, put the split peas, and water or stock. Bring to a boil, with the lid slightly uncovered. Lower flame and simmer until the peas begin to soften, about 30 minutes.

2. Add the ham hock, bacon, or pancetta, if using. Return to a boil. Lower flame and continue cooking until the peas begin to fall apart, about another 30 to 40 minutes.

3. If the squash is not organic, peel it. Cut in half and remove the seeds; scoop them out with a spoon, then either discard or roast them (see Note). Cut the squash into 1-inch chunks.

4. Add the squash chunks, onions, garlic, celery, and potato to the cooking peas. Return to a boil, covered. Lower flame and continue cooking until the squash has softened, about 20 minutes.

5. In a small bowl, dilute the miso in a ladle of soup broth. Return to the pot and season with the herbal sea salt and pepper. Add the butter and allow it to melt. Mix well. Serve the soup hot in ceramic bowls, topped with a sprig of dill or parsley, and whole-grain crackers on the side.

Cooking Tip: Winter squash such as butternut or buttercup squash does not need to be peeled if it is organic. However, commercially grown squash is sometimes coated with wax to increase its storage life. If you are cooking with this kind, peel the squash.

Note: To roast the seeds, preheat the oven to 350 degrees. Place the seeds in a bowl of water and clean off the squash fibers. Remove the seeds to a colander and drain. On an ungreased or parchment-lined baking pan, spread the seeds out evenly. (For salted seeds, sprinkle with salt.) Bake until golden brown, about 15 minutes, stirring about every 5 minutes to keep them from burning. Remove from the oven and cool. Store in a covered glass jar.

Nutritional Stars: Vitamin A, vitamin C, folic acid, zinc

 # Vegetable Stock au Bouquet Garni

Yield: 4 quarts stock   100% vegetarian

The bouquet garni:

3 to 4 sprigs fresh parsley, ends trimmed and washed
2 sprigs fresh or 1 teaspoon dried thyme (optional)
1 leek, split and washed (see page 31)
1 bay leaf
   Several celery ribs, preferably from the outer portion (optional)

The stock:

6 to 8 cups of any combination of fresh vegetables (see Note)
4 quarts purified water (enough to cover the vegetables by at least 1 inch)
¼ cup green lentils, sorted and washed
3 to 6 coriander seeds (optional)
2 tomatoes, chopped, or 2 teaspoons cider vinegar
5 black peppercorns
½ teaspoon celery seed
   Pinch cayenne pepper

(Vegetable Stock au Bouquet Garni—Continued)

The bouquet garni:

Bunch the parsley, thyme, leek, and bay leaf together and tie them with white cooking twine or place the herbs inside the celery ribs and bind the package together tightly with the twine.

The stock:

1. In a large stockpot, place the vegetables and/or peelings, water, lentils, coriander seeds, tomatoes or vinegar, peppercorns, celery seed, and cayenne. Add the bouquet garni. Bring to a boil with the lid slightly uncovered.

2. Once the pot has come to a boil, reduce the flame and simmer for 1 hour.

3. Turn off the flame and uncover, allowing the stock to sit and cool for at least 10 minutes.

4. Place a colander in a large bowl or another pot, and place in the sink (to allow for easier pouring). Carefully pour the stock into the colander. Set aside to drain completely and to allow the stock to settle.

5. Discard the vegetables and the garni.

6. The stock is now ready for immediate use. If the stock is to be stored, allow it to cool completely and then pour into containers. (Use plastic containers for freezer storage.) Label them with the type of stock and date. Refrigerate or freeze.

Cooking Tip: When making a vegetable stock, do not use cruciferous vegetables, such as cabbage, broccoli, cauliflower, and Brussels sprouts. These vegetables have a strong taste that can overpower your stock.

Note: Use a mixture of vegetables or a single kind, such as acorn, buttercup, or butternut squash, carrots, celeriac (celery root), celery stalks with leaves, garlic, leeks, onions, parsnips, and/or parsley root. The vegetables used can be cut into large pieces. If the vegetable skins have a wax covering or are nonorganic, and have possibly been sprayed with chemicals, peel them. You can also use vegetable peels and trimmings, such as corncobs, onion and garlic skins, potato skins, and winter squash seeds. The stock will be sweeter-tasting if the vegetables are organic.

Light Fish Stock

Yield: 4 to 6 quarts stock

1 to 2 pounds white fish bones and heads, including cod, scrod, red
    snapper, catfish, flounder, or sole
4 quarts purified water (or enough to cover the bones by at least
    1 inch)
2 tomatoes, chopped, or 2 teaspoons cider vinegar
3 or 4 allspice berries or white peppercorns
1 bay leaf
  Peel from ½ orange or lemon, preferably organic

1. In a large stockpot, place the fish bones and heads, water, tomatoes or vinegar, allspice or peppercorns, bay leaf, and orange or lemon peel. Bring to a boil with the lid slightly uncovered. Skim any discolored foam from the top and discard. Reduce flame and simmer, covered, for 45 to 60 minutes.

2. Turn off the flame and uncover, allowing the stock to sit and cool for at least 10 minutes.

3. Place a colander in a large bowl or another pot, and place in the sink (to allow for easier pouring). Carefully pour the stock into the colander. Set aside to drain completely and to allow the stock to settle. Discard the bones.

4. The stock is now ready for immediate use. If the stock is to be stored, allow it to cool completely and then pour into containers. (Use plastic containers for freezer storage.) Label them with the type of stock and date. Refrigerate or freeze.

Cooking Tip: Shrimp, clam, and lobster shells make excellent light-tasting stocks. Salmon, mackerel, tuna, and halibut—oilier types of fish, which have a stronger flavor—are not preferred for stocks.

Beef Bone or Poultry Stock

Yield: 4 quarts stock

2 to 3 pounds uncooked beef bones or 1 to 2 pounds uncooked or
    cooked chicken, turkey, or duck bones (see Note)
4 quarts purified water (enough to cover the bones and/or vegetables
    by at least 1 inch)
2 teaspoons cider vinegar or 2 tomatoes, chopped
3 or 4 black or white peppercorns (optional)
1 onion, peeled and stuck with 2 or 3 whole cloves
1 bay leaf
   Pinch paprika (optional)

1. In a large stockpot, place the beef or poultry bones, water, vinegar or tomatoes, peppercorns, onion, bay leaf, and paprika. Bring to a boil with the lid slightly
uncovered. Skim any discolored foam from the top and discard. Reduce flame and
simmer, covered, for 1½ hours.

2. Turn off the flame and uncover, allowing the stock to sit and cool for at least 10
minutes.

3. Place a colander in a large bowl or another pot, and place in the sink (to allow
for easier pouring). Carefully pour the stock into the colander. Set aside to drain
completely and to allow the stock to settle.

4. Remove any meat from the bones, and discard the bones (or give to your
favorite dog).

5. The stock is now ready for immediate use. If the stock is to be stored, allow it
to cool completely and then pour into containers. (Use plastic containers for freezer
storage.) Label them with the type of stock and date. Refrigerate or freeze.

Cooking Tip: Mature vegetables and meat from older animals are the most
flavorful for making stocks.

Note: For beef stock: Use meaty beef bones such as shanks, neck, knuckle, leg,
and/or oxtails. If the bones are too big, ask your butcher to cut them. For poultry
stock: We like to use backs, necks, feet, gizzards, and/or a carcass

---

Stock Variations with a Chicken Dinner

You can boil a whole chicken and eat it as is, or use the meat to make a salad, or slice it for sandwiches. You can also use the boiling liquid later as a stock. Here are some variations:

- **Chicken Noodle Soup:** Heat the stock and add a handful of whole wheat vermicelli noodles. Cook until tender and season with herbal sea salt.
- **Egg Drop Soup:** Heat the stock, bringing it to a boil. Season with herbal sea salt. In a small bowl, whisk 1 or 2 eggs. Drizzle the eggs into the hot soup while it's still cooking, just before serving.
- **Lemon Soup:** To the hot stock, add the juice of ½ to 1 fresh lemon (2 to 4 tablespoons) just before serving.
- **Garlic Soup:** Peel and mince 4 to 10 cloves garlic, add to the simmering stock, and cook for just a minute.
- **Mexican Garlic Soup:** Prepare the stock with garlic as above. Ladle the soup into large bowls and crack an egg into each. The hot soup will cook the egg just enough. Serve with lime wedges on the side.
- **Chicken Soup with Greens:** Heat the stock and add a small bunch of washed and chopped greens, such as kale, collards, spinach, or chard. Cook until tender and season with herbal sea salt.

 # Cajun Red Lentil and Corn Stew

Yield: 4 to 6 servings   100% vegetarian

The piquant flavors of Cajun spices make dishes such as this easy to like for those who are less familiar with vegetarian foods. The beans add a rich protein base to the corn rounds and other vegetables. A very satisfying and filling dish—and good for all.

PMS Benefits: Corn contains zinc, which facilitates the use of vitamin B6 (pyridoxine). B6 plays many roles in relation to PMS, stabilizing moods, preventing abdominal bloating, and reducing sugar cravings.

(Cajun Red Lentil and Corn Stew—Continued)
Before you begin, cook a pot of brown rice or use another leftover grain.

2 **cups red lentils, sorted and washed**
4 **cups homemade salt-free vegetable stock or purified water**
1 **bay leaf**
2 **large tomatoes, cores removed, chopped**
2 **onions, chopped**
2 **stalks celery, ends trimmed, chopped**
2 **cloves garlic, minced**
1 **parsnip, ends trimmed, chopped**
1 **red bell pepper, seeded and chopped**
1 **green bell pepper, seeded and chopped**
½ **teaspoon dried thyme**
½ **teaspoon ground mustard**
¼ **teaspoon ground pepper**
⅛ **teaspoon ground ginger**
2 **ears fresh corn, husks removed**
8 **sprigs fresh parsley, washed and thick stems removed**
3 **tablespoons unsalted butter, preferably organic, or**
   extra-virgin olive oil
2 **tablespoons lemon juice**
1½ **teaspoons herbal sea salt**
2 **cups cooked brown rice, hot or at room temperature**

1. In a large soup pot, bring the lentils, stock or water, and bay leaf to a boil, covered. Lower flame and simmer 10 minutes.

2. Add the tomatoes, onions, celery, garlic, parsnip, red and green peppers, thyme, mustard, pepper, and ginger. Return to a boil, reduce flame, and continue cooking for another 10 to 15 minutes, covered. Stir occasionally.

3. Cut the corn into 1-inch rounds. Add to the stew and stir well. Cover and cook until tender, 3 to 4 minutes.

4. Mince 4 sprigs of the parsley and add to the stew with the butter or olive oil, lemon juice, and herbal sea salt. Stir to combine thoroughly.

5. Place the cooked rice on a large, deep platter. Spoon the stew on top. Garnish with the remaining 4 sprigs of parsley.

Cooking Tip: Before they are cooked, red lentils start out crimson-red. Don't be surprised—as they cook, they lose their color and turn yellow-ocher.

Nutritional Stars: Vitamin B6, folic acid

Three-Bean Vegetarian Cassoulet

Yield: 6 servings   100% vegetarian

The flavors of a traditional cassoulet draw on the spices and fats of sausages and other meats. To replace them without losing flavor, we've added fennel and sage, lots of hearty and tasty vegetables, and topped the pot with a nutty bread-crumb mixture that is baked until golden.

PMS Benefits: Reduce the amount of meat and dairy foods in your diet to avoid PMS symptoms, and include more beans and peas. These plant foods are good sources of low-fat and high-quality protein.

Before you begin, soak ¼ cup *each,* sorted and washed, dried cannellini, navy, and Great Northern beans in three bowls with 2 cups purified water in each bowl for 6 hours or overnight.

½ **cup soaked cannellini beans (from ¼ cup dried beans)**
½ **cup soaked navy beans (from ¼ cup dried beans)**
½ **cup soaked Great Northern beans (from ¼ cup dried beans)**
1 **bay leaf**
1 **teaspoon dried or 2 sprigs fresh rosemary**
1 **teaspoon dried or 2 sprigs fresh marjoram**
6 **tablespoons unsalted butter, preferably organic**
2 **onions, chopped**
3 **cloves garlic, minced**
1 **teaspoon dried sage**
1 **teaspoon fennel seeds**
2 **carrots, ends trimmed, chopped**
2 **turnips, ends trimmed, chopped**
2 **parsnips, ends trimmed, chopped**
2 **stalks celery, ends trimmed, chopped**
1 **teaspoon herbal sea salt**
¼ **teaspoon ground white pepper**
1 **bunch collard greens or kale, ends trimmed, washed, and chiffonade-cut (see Cooking Tip 1) or chopped**
½ **cup whole-grain bread crumbs**
½ **cup almonds, chopped fine**
¼ **teaspoon sea salt**
   Pinch ground black pepper

(Three-Bean Vegetarian Cassoulet—Continued)

1. With your hands or a slotted spoon, remove each batch of soaked beans from the soaking water and put into three separate saucepans. Add 2 cups fresh water to each pot. To each pot, add one of the herbs: the bay leaf, rosemary, and marjoram, using all three. Bring to a boil, covered, lower flame, and simmer for 30 minutes (see Cooking Tip 2).

2. In a Dutch oven, on the stovetop, heat 3 tablespoons butter and add the onions, garlic, sage, and fennel seeds and stir well. Cook on a medium flame until the onions begin to brown, about 10 minutes. Stir frequently.

3. Stir the carrots, turnips, parsnips, and celery into the onion mixture. Cook uncovered for 3 to 4 minutes. Stir occasionally.

4. Place a colander in a bowl and drain all three pots of the beans, reserving the liquid. Remove the bay leaf and fresh herb stems, if used, and discard. Add the beans to the onion mixture. Stir well. Add half the reserved bean liquid to the mixture, covering it about three-fourths. Bring to a boil, covered. Lower flame and simmer for 30 minutes. (Save the remaining liquid for soup or use as a stock.)

5. Adjust the oven shelves to fit the Dutch oven. Preheat the oven to 375 degrees.

6. Season the bean mixture with herbal sea salt and white pepper, and stir well. Stir in the collards or kale and cook uncovered for 4 or 5 minutes.

7. In a small skillet or saucepan, melt the remaining 3 tablespoons butter. Remove from heat and add the bread crumbs, almonds, sea salt, and black pepper. Mix well. Sprinkle the crumb mixture over the beans.

8. Place the cassoulet in the preheated oven. Bake uncovered until the top is golden, 20 to 30 minutes.

9. Place a trivet on the table and put the Dutch oven on it. Add a serving spoon to spoon into wide, shallow bowls. Serve with whole-grain noodles or hearty bread chunks and a salad on the side.

Cooking Tip 1: To chiffonade, remove the thick stem from the greens and discard. Lay three or four leaves on top of one another. Starting from the broad part of the leaf, tightly roll the stack of leaves into a thick cigar shape. With one hand hold the roll, and using a chef's knife, slice the greens into very thin strips. As they are cut from the roll, they will begin to unravel. The strips can be cut crosswise, if you prefer shorter pieces.

Cooking Tip 2: It is preferable to cook the beans in separate pots since they all have slightly different cooking times; this also keeps the flavors of the beans and herbs more distinct.

Nutritional Stars: Vitamin A, B-complex vitamins, vitamin E, vitamin C, folic acid, magnesium, copper, iron, manganese, omega-3 fatty acids

Four-Onion and Red-Bean Vegetable Tagine

Yield: 6 servings   100% vegetarian

This Moroccan stew is made traditionally in a clay pot and left to cook slowly all day. After eating this dish, you may find yourself buying tickets to Marrakech!

PMS Benefits: You're not only what you eat. You are what you absorb. If you make a special effort to consume all the nutrients that quiet PMS, you still need a healthy digestive tract to benefit from them. A normally functioning digestive tract requires fiber to provide bulk. Whole grains, beans, vegetables, and fruits supply plenty of fiber to move digested foods through the intestines.

Before you begin, soak 1 cup sorted and washed dried kidney or pinto beans in a bowl with 5 cups purified water for 6 hours or overnight.

      2 **cups soaked kidney or pinto beans (from 1 cup dried beans)**
      3 **cups homemade salt-free vegetable stock or purified water**
    ½ **cup unsulphured sun-dried tomatoes or 4 fresh tomatoes, cores
          removed, chopped**
  1½ **teaspoons cumin**
      1 **teaspoon ginger**
    ½ **teaspoon turmeric**
    ½ **teaspoon paprika**
      1 **cinnamon stick or ½ teaspoon powdered cinnamon**
      2 **tablespoons unsalted butter, preferably organic, or extra-virgin olive oil**
      1 **yellow onion, sliced**
      1 **red onion, sliced**
      1 **white onion, sliced, or 2 leeks, split, washed, and chopped**
      2 **cloves garlic, minced**
      1 **carrot, ends trimmed, diced**
      1 **sweet potato or yam, peeled and diced**
      8 **pearl onions, peeled**
    ¼ **cup lemon juice, preferably fresh**
    ½ **teaspoon coriander powder**
    ½ **teaspoon ground pepper**
      1 **bunch fresh cilantro (coriander), washed, thick stems
          removed, minced**
      1 **teaspoon sea salt**
      1 **recipe Minted Couscous and Green Pea Timbales (see page 100)**
    10 **to 15 kalamata or other imported black olives**

(Four-Onion and Red-Bean Vegetable Tagine—Continued)

1. With your hands or a slotted spoon, remove the beans from the soaking water and put into a large pot with the stock or fresh water, tomatoes, cumin, ginger, turmeric, paprika, and cinnamon stick or powder. Bring to a boil, covered; lower heat and simmer for 30 minutes.

2. In a medium-sized skillet, on a moderate flame, heat the butter or olive oil. Sauté the yellow, red, and white onions or leeks uncovered until the edges begin to brown, about 10 minutes. Stir occasionally to prevent burning.

3. Add the garlic, carrot, sweet potato or yam, pearl onions, lemon juice, coriander powder, and pepper. Cook, stirring, 1 minute. Add ¼ cup bean cooking liquid to the onion mixture and cook for 1 more minute, stirring to deglaze the pan.

4. Add the vegetables to the beans and cover. Cook until the beans are soft, about another 20 minutes.

5. Stir in one-half of the cilantro and the sea salt. Cook another 1 to 2 minutes. Spoon tagine over the cooked Minted Couscous and Green Pea Timbales and garnish with the remaining cilantro and olives.

Cooking Tip: Olives can be stored for a long time if they are kept in brine (salted water) or covered in oil. Either way, store them in the refrigerator. If they are very salty, store them in purified water for one or two days to reduce their salinity.

Nutritional Stars: Vitamin B6, vitamin C, folic acid, iron, magnesium, manganese

Multi-Potato Stew with Beef and Lamb Cubes

Yield: 4 servings

Add any other favorite vegetables, such as turnips, daikon, burdock, or butternut squash for a hearty and homey meal.

PMS Benefits: Salt can lead to fluid retention and menstrual bloating. We cook with small amounts of sea salt, as in this recipe, and rely on savory flavorings for the flavor accent.

½ **cup whole-grain flour, such as whole wheat or high-lysine corn**
½ **teaspoon sea salt**
¼ **teaspoon ground pepper**
½ **pound beef, preferably organic, cubed**
½ **pound lamb, preferably organic, cubed**
2 **to 4 tablespoons extra-virgin olive oil or unsalted butter, preferably organic**

1 onion, chopped
2 to 4 cloves garlic, minced
3 to 4 cups purified water or homemade salt-free stock
3 stalks celery, ends trimmed, chopped
2 carrots, ends trimmed, chopped
1 bay leaf
1 teaspoon dried rosemary or thyme
2 small Yukon gold or red potatoes
4 to 8 Peruvian blue potatoes
4 to 8 fingerling potatoes
   Sprigs fresh parsley, optional

1. In a medium-sized bowl, combine the flour, salt, and pepper. Drop a few cubes of meat into the flour and coat evenly. Remove to a plate and continue with the other cubes until all have been coated.

2. In a large Dutch oven, on a medium flame, heat 2 tablespoons oil or butter. Add a single layer of meat cubes without crowding them. Brown on all sides, turning with a fork or tongs. If needed, brown the cubes in two batches. Add oil or butter as needed. Remove all of the browned meat cubes to a plate.

3. To the same pot, add the onion, garlic, and any remaining flour. Cook, stirring, on medium-high heat for 2 or 3 minutes, being careful not to let burn.

4. Return the meat to the pot and add the water or stock, celery, carrots, bay leaf, and rosemary or thyme. Cover and bring to a boil. Lower heat and simmer until the meat cubes are almost tender, about 30 minutes.

5. Add the unpeeled Yukon gold or red, Peruvian blue, and fingerling potatoes. Cover and continue to cook until the potatoes have softened, another 15 minutes.

6. Season with additional salt and pepper, as desired, and stir one last time. Remove the bay leaf. Using a large spoon, scoop the stew into a beautiful ceramic serving bowl. Top with a few sprigs of fresh parsley, if desired.

Cooking Tip: Cut the larger potatoes into pieces, so that all of the potatoes are about equal size. Do not peel them for this recipe.

Note: This can be prepared without meat, using additional vegetables. Begin with step 3.

Nutritional Stars: B-complex vitamins, copper, iron, magnesium, manganese, selenium, zinc

Sweet Potato and Turnip Stew with Chicken Strips

Yield: 4 servings

Savory and sweet, this stew will dampen your craving for something more after you've finished a meal. The potatoes and turnips are full of rich minerals and the chicken has protein with just a little fat—all needed to stop the PMS munchies. Make a batch and serve it with whole-grain pasta, brown rice, or over toast.

PMS Benefits: Sweet potatoes contain vitamins A and E, two nutrients that help relieve swollen and tender breasts sometimes associated with PMS.

½ cup whole-grain flour, such as whole wheat or high-lysine corn
½ teaspoon sea salt
¼ teaspoon ground pepper
1 pound boneless chicken breasts, cut into strips
2 to 4 tablespoons extra-virgin olive oil, unsalted butter, preferably
    organic, or ghee (see page 227)
1 onion, chopped
2 to 4 cloves garlic, minced
3 to 4 cups purified water or homemade salt-free stock
3 stalks celery, ends trimmed, chopped
2 carrots, ends trimmed, chopped
1 sweet potato or yam, peeled and cut into large chunks
1 or 2 turnips, ends trimmed, cut into chunks
6-inch piece daikon, cut into chunks
1 bay leaf
1 teaspoon dried basil or tarragon
1 bunch watercress, spinach, chard, or arugula, washed and chopped
    coarsely
    Sprigs fresh parsley (optional)

1. In a medium-sized bowl, combine the flour, salt, and pepper. Drop a few strips of chicken into the flour and coat evenly. Remove to a plate and continue with the other strips until all have been coated.

2. In a large Dutch oven, on a medium flame, heat the oil, butter, or ghee. Add a single layer of chicken strips without crowding. Brown on all sides, turning with a fork or tongs. If needed, brown the strips in two batches. Add oil or butter as needed. Remove the browned chicken to a plate.

3. To the same pot, add the onion, garlic, and any remaining flour. Cook, stirring, on medium-high heat for 2 or 3 minutes. Be careful not to let burn.

4. Add the water or stock, celery, carrots, sweet potato or yam, turnips, daikon, bay leaf, and basil or tarragon. Cover and bring to a boil. Lower heat and simmer until the chicken and vegetables are soft, 30 to 45 minutes.

5. Add the chopped greens, season with additional salt and pepper if desired, and stir. Cover and cook on low heat until the greens wilt, 4 to 5 minutes. Stir one last time.

6. Using a large spoon, scoop the stew into a beautiful ceramic serving bowl. Top with a few sprigs of fresh parsley if desired, and serve with a side of noodles or brown rice.

Cooking Tip: What most of us consider to be yams, the sweet, orange-fleshed tubers common in our own supermarkets, are actually sweet potatoes. True yams are grown in the tropics and subtropics and have a brown or rusty-tan color and a textured outer surface. Yams are shaped like a log, and the interior is mucilaginous and either white, ivory, or yellow. The taste is not at all what we are accustomed to. Yams can be bland, nutty-tasting, or have virtually no taste at all.

Note: This can be made without meat. Begin with step 3.

Nutritional Stars: Vitamin A, B-complex vitamins, vitamin C, vitamin E

A Bowl Full

Raw and Cooked Salads

Dressings

Dips and Spreads

Salad as a Meal

A salad can be a lot more than a bowl full of iceberg lettuce. You will discover a cornucopia of additional ingredients in your grocery store. Salad greens with red tips, strong, sturdy green points, fluted bunches, and buttery soft leaves decorate the bins. Begin with romaine, spinach, escarole, chicory, watercress, and mesclun leaves, then accompany them with red or green cabbage, radishes, and fresh herbs, sliced onion or chives, and sprouts. Add nuts and seeds, and you've got a magnificent dinner salad.

To make a salad into a meal, look for filling ingredients that will satisfy your protein needs. Mix a grain salad with a bean dressing or serve with whole-grain bread and a side of bean spread. Add some cooked fish or chicken to a green salad, or start with a fresh bean salad and add whole-grain bread with a smear of organic butter. If you are not troubled by cramps, you can also add hard-boiled eggs, an excellent protein source. Garnish your salad with cherry tomatoes, cucumber slices, olives, walnuts, green and red pepper slices, and serve with whole-grain crackers or bread sticks. Have fun experimenting with the color of grated carrots or beets, the texture of thinly sliced red cabbage, and the flavors of fresh herbs!

Louisiana Multicolored Slaw with Caraway Seeds

Yield: 2 to 2½ quarts   100% vegetarian

It's hard to make a small amount of slaw, but the great news is that it tastes better as it ages—and lasts for more than a week when it's prepared without mayonnaise, as we do here.

PMS Benefits: Vitamin C fights emotional stress and reduces fatigue. It promotes a healthy immune system, aids in the absorption of iron, and eases heavy monthly bleeding when combined with flavonoids. Cabbage contains both vitamin C and flavonoids.

¼ head green cabbage, core removed, sliced thin
¼ head red cabbage, core removed, sliced thin
1 yellow onion, sliced thin or grated
1 red onion, sliced thin or grated

(Louisiana Multicolored Slaw with Caraway Seeds—Continued)

    2 **teaspoons sea salt**
    1 **carrot, ends trimmed, grated**
    1 **cucumber, peeled, seeded, and grated**
    4 **red radishes, ends trimmed, grated or minced**
    1 **bunch parsley, thick stems removed, washed and minced**
    2 **sprigs fresh dill, thick stems removed, washed and minced**
    2 **sprigs fresh cilantro (coriander), thick stems removed,
       washed and minced**
    1 **teaspoon caraway seeds**
   ½ **cup unsulphured currants**
    1 **recipe A Basic Dressing (see page 60) or Yogurt Herb Dressing
       (see page 62) (see Note)**

1. In a large bowl, put the green and red cabbages, yellow and red onions, and sea salt. With your hands, toss the salad fixings together, rubbing and squeezing them until the cabbage begins to release its liquid and soften, 1 or 2 minutes. If this is not done the cabbage is hard to chew (see Cooking Tip). Set aside for 5 minutes.

2. Place a colander in the sink. Pour in the cabbage mixture and allow the liquid to drain. Taste a piece of cabbage and if it is too salty, rinse one-half of the cabbage mixture under cold water. Shake the colander and press the cabbage to drain the liquid very well.

3. Put the cabbage into a large, clean mixing bowl. Add the carrot, cucumber, radishes, parsley, dill, cilantro, and caraway, and mix well. Toss in the currants and pour the dressing of choice over the cabbage and mix. Taste and add additional salt and pepper, if desired. Refrigerate the slaw at least 15 minutes or overnight, if time permits. Toss again just before serving, and garnish.

Cooking Tip: Keep your salad dressing from becoming too watery by salting the cabbage and rubbing its leaves between your hands—this softens and tenderizes the cabbage and helps to release its liquids.

Note: Deciding on which salad dressing you use is a matter of consistency: A Basic Dressing is a clear vinaigrette, and the Yogurt Herb Dressing is like mayonnaise.

Nutritional Stars: Vitamin A, vitamin C, folic acid

Quick Greek Salad

Yield: 4 servings   100% vegetarian

Serve this quick-to-make salad with whole-grain crackers and our Chickpea and Red Onion Hummus (see page 63) or a ready-made bean spread from the supermarket. You can't beat this combination.

PMS Benefits: Vitamin C aids in tissue growth and repair, and helps you to withstand menstrual stress. Vitamin C is found in vegetables such as fresh peppers, tomatoes, and parsley.

2 **ripe tomatoes, cores removed, or ½ pint cherry tomatoes**
1 **red or yellow bell pepper, seeded**
1 **red or Vidalia onion, peeled**
1 **cup crumbled imported feta cheese**
4 **sprigs fresh parsley, washed, thick stems removed, and chopped
    coarsely**
½ **teaspoon dried Greek oregano**
8 **to 10 Greek olives**
1 **recipe A Basic Dressing (see page 60)**

1. Cut the tomatoes into bite-sized pieces or the cherry tomatoes in half. Put them in an oversized serving bowl. Cut the pepper into slices and then cut across in half or thirds. Slice or dice the onion. Add to the tomatoes with the feta, parsley, oregano, and olives.

2. Toss the vegetables with the dressing and serve with a side of hummus and whole-grain crackers or chunks of bread.

Cooking Tip: Forgot to buy the hummus? Add some protein and fiber to your salad by tossing in some cooked beans.

Nutritional Stars: B-complex vitamins, vitamin C, omega-3 fatty acids

Cauliflower Salad with Currants, Anchovies, and Pine Nuts

Yield: 6 servings

Remove the anchovies from this yummy cooked vegetable salad, and you've got a 100% vegetarian meal.

PMS Benefits: Potassium benefits a woman's health by helping maintain a regular heartbeat and a healthy nervous system. It also helps to regulate the body's water balance. Deficiencies in this important mineral can cause sodium retention, PMS swelling, and edema. Potassium-rich foods include currants, pine nuts, and anchovies.

 1 **head cauliflower, core removed, and washed**
 1 **cup purified water**
 ¼ **cup extra-virgin olive oil**
 ¼ **cup cider or brown rice vinegar**
 1 **tablespoon prepared mustard**
    Pinch sea salt (optional)
    Several grinds fresh white pepper
 4 **to 6 fresh flat anchovies or anchovy fillets packed in olive oil,**
       drained (optional)
 4 **to 6 sprigs fresh parsley, washed, thick stems removed, and minced**
 3 **scallions, ends trimmed, minced**
 ¼ **cup unsulphured currants**
 ¼ **cup pine nuts**

1. Using a paring knife, separate the cauliflower into individual, bite-sized florets and put it into a large saucepan with the water. (A steamer basket can be used, if preferred.) Cover and bring to a boil on a high flame. Reduce heat and simmer until the cauliflower is tender when a fork is inserted, 7 to 10 minutes. When cooked, remove the cauliflower with a slotted spoon to a large serving bowl.

2. In a small bowl, mix together the olive oil, vinegar, mustard, salt, if using, and pepper. Pour over the cauliflower and toss. Chop the anchovies, if using, and add with the parsley, scallions, and currants. Stir again.

3. Heat a small skillet on a medium flame and toast the pine nuts, stirring continuously to keep the nuts from burning. Cook until a light golden brown, 3 to 4 minutes. Immediately sprinkle on the salad (removing the nuts from the pan keeps them from burning).

4. Serve as is or allow the salad to marinate 15 minutes before serving. (Remove leftover vegetable salads from the refrigerator at least 15 minutes before serving, to allow the flavors to warm slightly.) Toss the salad again and serve.

Cooking Tip: Use anchovies within a day; otherwise their flavor will become strong and unpleasant.

Nutritional Stars: Vitamin C, potassium, omega-3 fatty acids

 # Grated Kohlrabi, Jícama, and Daikon Salad with Sesame Seeds

Yield: 6 servings   100% vegetarian

Here is a variation on the familiar theme of slaw. Just replace the cabbage with these easy-to-find vegetables that may be new to you, but which are very healthy and taste delicious raw.

PMS Benefits: Sesame seeds are rich in many important PMS nutrients, including vitamins B, B2, B3, B5, B6, C, and E, and the minerals copper, iron, magnesium, and zinc.

- 1 **large kohlrabi, ends trimmed, grated**
- 1 **jícama, peeled and grated**
- 1 **carrot, ends trimmed, grated**
- ½ **daikon radish, grated**
- 1 **recipe Thai Lime-Ginger Dressing (see page 61) or Creamy Balsamic Almond-Butter Dressing (see page 62)**
- ¼ **cup raw unhulled brown or black sesame seeds**
- 2 **or 3 sprigs fresh parsley, washed and stems trimmed short**

1. In a large bowl, mix together the grated kohlrabi, jícama, carrot, and daikon. Pour the dressing of your choosing over the vegetables and mix well. Transfer the salad to a serving bowl and set aside.

2. In a small, heavy-bottomed saucepan, on medium-high heat, dry-roast the sesame seeds, stirring constantly. The seeds will begin to pop, and some may jump out of the pot. Keep stirring until they smell fragrant and toasty, about 3 minutes. Make sure to move the seeds constantly to keep them from burning.

3. Pour the hot seeds over the grated salad and top with several sprigs of parsley. Serve and enjoy.

(Grated Kohlrabi, Jicama, and Daikon Salad with Sesame Seeds—Continued)
    Cooking Tip: Use a food processor with a grater attachment to prepare this salad quickly.
    Nutritional Stars: Vitamin A, B-complex vitamins, vitamin C, calcium, copper, iron, magnesium, zinc

 # Broccoli Salad with Red Onion and Black Olives

Yield: 6 servings   100% vegetarian

Add beans, grains, hard-cooked eggs, nuts, or seeds to this simple salad for a more filling protein combination.

PMS Benefits: Appreciable amounts of vitamin A are found in green foods such as broccoli, as well as parsley, scallions, asparagus, and many leafy greens such as bok choy, kale, spinach, and collards. Try this recipe if you feel bloated or fatigued.

   1 **bunch broccoli, washed (see Note)**
   1 **cup purified water**
   8 **to 10 olives, pitted and chopped**
   2 **cloves garlic, minced**
   1 **red onion, sliced thin**
  ¼ **cup reconstituted unsulphured sun-dried tomatoes, chopped**
  ¼ **cup fresh lemon juice**
   3 **tablespoons extra-virgin olive oil**
   2 **tablespoons flaxseed oil**
  ½ **teaspoon dried oregano**
  ½ **teaspoon herbal sea salt**
    Several grinds fresh pepper

    1. With a paring knife, remove the florets of the broccoli and cut into medium-sized pieces. Set aside. Remove the leaves and chop coarsely. Trim the fibrous outer layer of the stalks and discard. Cut the stalks into diagonal slices or sticks and toss with the leaves.
    2. In a large saucepan, bring the water to a boil. Add the broccoli stems and leaves. (A steamer basket can be used, if preferred.) Cover and bring back to a boil, then reduce heat and simmer for 5 minutes. Add the florets and continue cooking until the broccoli is tender when pierced with a fork and bright green. Total cooking time is 7 to 10 minutes.

3. Using a slotted spoon, remove the broccoli to a serving bowl and toss with the olives, garlic, onion, and tomatoes.

4. In a small bowl, mix together the lemon juice, olive and flaxseed oils, oregano, herbal sea salt, and pepper. Pour over the broccoli and toss.

5. Serve as is or allow the salad to marinate 15 minutes before serving. (Remove leftover vegetable salads from the refrigerator at least 15 minutes before serving, to allow the flavors to warm slightly.)

Cooking Tip: Use a potato peeler to remove the tough outer layer from the broccoli stems. Then slice the stems and cook them for this salad.

Note: Substitute any of these vegetables for the broccoli: asparagus (tough ends removed), beets, black radish, bronzini Brussels sprouts, cabbage, carrots, cauliflower, corn kernels, daikon, fennel, green beans, kohlrabi, leeks, mushrooms, onions, potatoes, red and/or green peppers (seeded), snow peas, sugar snaps, sweet potato, turnips, yams, or any greens such as broccoli rabe, kale, collards, or turnip greens.

Nutritional Stars: Vitamin A, B-complex vitamins, vitamin C

 # Phyto Rice and Quinoa Salad

Yield: 4 servings   100% vegetarian

A variation on the theme of a single-grain salad, this one incorporates two grains— brown rice and quinoa (keen-wa), a staple of the ancient civilizations of the Andes. You can use leftover cooked grain to speed up the salad-making.

PMS Benefits: The whole grains of this recipe contain fiber, B vitamins, and protein, and by adding quinoa, you broaden the variety of ingredients that make up your meals. A basic tenet of good health, this increases the likelihood that you'll consume a full range of nutrients.

½ **cup brown rice, washed (see page 85)**
½ **cup quinoa, millet, or amaranth, washed (see Note)**
2½ **cups purified water**
½ **teaspoon sea salt plus additional as needed**
2 **stalks celery, ends trimmed, minced**
3 **tablespoons extra-virgin olive oil**
2 **tablespoons flaxseed oil**
¼ **cup cider vinegar**

(Phyto Rice and Quinoa Salad—Continued)

  2 tablespoons lemon juice
10 to 20 snow peas or green beans, tips removed, cut into
      thirds diagonally
  1 green bell pepper, seeded and minced
  ½ **bunch parsley, washed, thick stems removed, and minced**
  ½ **bunch basil, leaves only, washed and cut into slivers**
  3 scallions, ends trimmed, chopped
  ½ **bunch chives or 3 additional scallions, minced**
  1 head Boston or Bibb lettuce, leaves separated and washed

1. In a medium-sized saucepan, put the rice, quinoa, 2 cups water, and salt. Bring to a boil, covered, reduce flame, and simmer for 55 minutes. For thin-bottomed pots or stoves that are hard to adjust to a very low flame, use a heat diffuser.

2. Using a fork, scratch the surface of the grains to fluff and separate grains. Pour into a large bowl. Add the celery, olive and flaxseed oils, vinegar, and lemon juice. Toss and set aside to cool and allow flavors to infuse, at least 15 minutes.

3. In a small pot, bring the remaining ½ cup water to a boil. Add the snow peas or green beans, cover, and steam (30 seconds for snow peas or 3 minutes for green beans). Place a colander in the sink and pour the snow peas in. Run cold water over them to stop the cooking process.

4. To assemble the salad: Add the snow peas or green beans to the cooled rice and quinoa mixture with the green pepper, parsley, basil, scallions, and chives. Taste and add more salt, if desired. Stir well.

5. Arrange one large or several small lettuce leaves on individual plates. Serve a scoop of salad on the leaves along with some bean spread and breadsticks for a complete protein. *Bon appétit!*

Cooking Tip: When two grains have different cooking times and they're being cooked together in the same saucepan, cook them according to the grain with the longest cooking time.

Note: You can substitute other cooked whole grains or pasta for the suggested grains in the recipe. Try barley, bulgur, couscous, soba (buckwheat) pasta, udon (whole wheat) pasta, and whole-grain pasta in various shapes (for example, penne, elbows, or fettuccini).

Nutritional Stars: B-complex vitamins, omega-3 fatty acids

Complete Meal Bulgur Salad

Yield: 4 servings   100% vegetarian

We love all-in-one-bowl dishes! In this nutrient-rich recipe, bulgur supplies the fiber, while eggs add valuable protein. If you have hard-cooked eggs on hand, you're ready to prepare this recipe.

PMS Benefits: A meal that contains carbohydrates, protein, and fat gives you a steady source of energy, since these foods break down at different rates. The bulgur in this recipe, a complex carbohydrate, provides fuel for the first hour and a half. The protein-rich eggs break down next and kick in as an energy source, and finally the fats in the walnuts, avocado, and olive oil break down and yield energy three hours after eating.

2 **cups purified water**
1 **cup whole-grain bulgur wheat**
½ **teaspoon sea salt plus additional as needed**
3 **tablespoons extra-virgin olive oil**
3 **tablespoons flaxseed oil**
6 **tablespoons fresh lemon juice**
2 **hard-cooked eggs, preferably organic, peeled and chopped**
4 **to 6 sprigs fresh cilantro (coriander) or parsley, washed, thick stems removed, and minced**
4 **to 6 springs fresh dill, washed, thick stems removed, minced**
½ **cup reconstituted unsulphured sun-dried tomatoes, chopped, or ½ pint cherry tomatoes, cut in half**
¼ **cup raw walnuts or pecans, chopped coarsely**
½ **head romaine lettuce, washed, chopped or cut in a chiffonade (see Cooking Tip 1, page 40) and spun dry**
1 **ripe avocado, cut in half, remove and discard pit**
4 **red radishes, ends trimmed**

1. In a medium-sized saucepan, covered, bring the water to a boil. Add the bulgur and salt. Return to a boil, covered, lower heat, and simmer for 10 minutes.

2. Using a fork, scratch the surface of the bulgur to fluff and pour into a large bowl. Add the olive and flaxseed oils and lemon juice. Stir well and set aside to cool.

3. To assemble the salad: Toss the eggs, cilantro, dill, tomatoes, and walnuts with the cooled bulgur.

(Complete Meal Bulgur Salad—Continued)

4. To serve: On large individual dishes, divide the romaine among the four plates. Scoop the Bulgur Salad on top of two-thirds of the lettuce. Cut the avocado into slices and place two or three slices alongside each salad on the remaining one-third lettuce. Add a radish to the side.

Cooking Tip: To reconstitute sun-dried tomatoes, place them in a saucepan, cover with water, and bring to a boil with the lid on. Turn off flame and allow them to soak until cool, 10 to 15 minutes.

Nutritional Stars: Vitamin A, B-complex vitamins, vitamin C, copper, iron, magnesium, omega-3 fatty acids

 # Chickpeas, Feta, and Roasted Sweet Red Pepper Salad

Yield: 4 servings   100% vegetarian

Here's a salad that travels well. Pack a serving for lunch on the job.

PMS Benefits: Chickpeas contain many minerals, including zinc, iron, copper, magnesium, and calcium, needed to support the intricate chemistry of your monthly cycle. Your body requires minerals for proper cell function and structure and to smooth utilization of vitamins and other nutrients.

Before you begin, soak 1 cup dried chickpeas in 5 cups purified water for 6 hours or overnight.

- 2 **cups soaked chickpeas (from 1 cup dried peas)**
- 4 **cups purified water**
- 2 **red bell peppers, core removed, seeded or ½ cup reconstituted**
    sun-dried tomatoes, chopped
    Sea salt
- ¼ **cup extra-virgin olive oil**
- 2 **tablespoons flaxseed oil**
- ¼ **cup cider vinegar or lemon juice**
    Ground pepper
- 3 **scallions, ends trimmed, chopped**
- ¼ **pound imported feta, crumbled**

1. With your hands or a slotted spoon, remove the chickpeas from the soaking water to a saucepan. Pour in the fresh water and bring to a boil, covered. Reduce flame and simmer 45 minutes.

2. Roast the peppers over a direct flame or under the broiler, turning after the skin has charred—every 1 to 2 minutes. When the entire pepper is black, remove from the heat and place in a covered bowl or paper bag. Set aside to cool at least 10 minutes. If using sun-dried tomatoes, slice them into strips and cut crosswise into bite-size pieces. Place in a small bowl and set aside.

3. Add the sea salt to the chickpeas, and continue to cook until soft, another 15 to 20 minutes.

4. Place a colander in a bowl. Clean the peppers over the colander to catch the juices. Remove the skins and discard. Slice the peppers into thin strips and then cut crosswise into bite-sized pieces. In a large serving bowl, mix together the pepper juices, chopped pepper or sun-dried tomatoes, olive and flaxseed oils, vinegar or lemon juice, salt, and pepper. Set aside.

5. Return the colander to the bowl and pour in the chickpeas. (Save the liquid for a soup or use as a stock.) Pour the well-drained beans into the marinating pepper mixture. Set aside to cool to room temperature.

6. Add the scallions and feta, and toss. Add additional salt and pepper as needed. Toss again before serving.

Cooking Tip: Purchase imported feta made with sheep or goat's milk instead of cow's milk for a low-fat cheese with a better taste. Store it in a container filled with purified water and change the water weekly. If the cheese is too salty for your taste, change the water more frequently to decrease the salinity.

Nutritional Stars: Vitamin C, calcium, copper, iron, magnesium, zinc

Here are more suggestions for colorful bean salads:

Black beans: red pepper bits, corn kernels
Navy beans: brown rice, chopped scallions, sun-dried tomato bits
Pinto beans: cannellini beans, fresh parsley, white onion
Great Northern beans: cilantro, cherry tomatoes, chopped scallions
Black-eyed peas: lima beans, grated carrot, yellow onion
Chickpeas: steamed broccoli, chopped shallots, roasted red pepper slices,
            minced garlic
Cannellini beans: red onion, fresh dill, steamed sugar snaps

Salad Dressings—Understanding the Basics

A basic salad dressing is made up of a **sour** element and a **fatty** element. The sour portion can be lemon or lime juice, or any kind of vinegar, such as cider or brown rice. Choose a good-quality fat, such as extra-virgin olive oil, flaxseed oil, nut butter, yogurt, sour cream, or buttermilk. Then embellish these two basics with **flavor enhancers** like sea salt or herbal sea salt, ground black or white pepper, dried or fresh herbs, spices, mustard, onion, garlic, apple juice, or honey.

Once you know the basic proportions for salad dressing, it is easy to create any flavor. Try 1 part oil to 1 part lemon or vinegar, and salt to taste. If you prefer a less tart taste, just reduce the vinegar or add a little more oil. Other flavorings are usually added in ½ to 2 teaspoon proportions. Mix the ingredients well and your homemade dressing is ready to use. (See "Understanding and Knowing Your Ingredients" in the Appendix, on page 225, for information on mayonnaise and ketchup.) We've developed A Basic Dressing to give you the idea—have a ball!

A Basic Dressing

Yield: 1 cup   100% vegetarian

  5 **to 6 tablespoons extra-virgin olive oil**
  3 **tablespoons flaxseed oil or additional extra-virgin olive oil**
  ½ **cup lemon juice or cider vinegar**
  1 **tablespoon prepared mustard**
  ¼ **to ½ teaspoon dried basil, oregano, or marjoram**
  ¼ **teaspoon herbal sea salt**
  1 **or 2 pinches ground pepper**

1. In a jar or blender, mix 5 tablespoons olive oil with the flaxseed oil, lemon juice, mustard, herb of choice, herbal sea salt, and pepper. Shake or blend well.

2. With a carrot stick or a lettuce leaf, taste the dressing. If it is too sour, add the additional 1 tablespoon olive oil.

3. Store leftover dressing in a glass jar in the refrigerator. Shake before using.

Cooking Tip: Mustard helps to emulsify dressings and keeps them from separating.

Thai Lime-Ginger Dressing

Yield: 1 cup   100% vegetarian

1 1-inch piece fresh ginger, grated
¼ cup lime or lemon juice, preferably fresh
¼ cup unsweetened pineapple or apple juice
2 tablespoons flaxseed oil
2 tablespoons extra-virgin olive oil
3 tablespoons imported soy sauce
2 cloves garlic, minced fine
1 to 2 pinches sea salt
3 sprigs fresh cilantro (coriander), washed, thick stems removed,
     and chopped coarsely
3 sprigs fresh mint, washed, thick stems removed, and chopped
     coarsely

1. In a jar or blender, mix together the ginger, lime or lemon juice, pineapple or apple juice, flaxseed and olive oils, soy sauce, garlic, and sea salt. Mix well.

2. Add the cilantro and mint and pour over the salad and toss.

3. Store leftover dressing in a glass jar in the refrigerator. Shake before using.

Cooking Tip: Specialty cooking stores carry a grater designed especially for ginger that breaks up the fibers into smaller pieces, yielding more flavor.

Yogurt Herb Dressing

Yield: 1 cup   100% vegetarian

½ cup plain yogurt with active cultures, preferably organic
1 to 2 tablespoons cider vinegar or lemon juice
2 to 4 tablespoons purified water
½ teaspoon powdered mustard
¼ to ½ teaspoon sea salt
1 to 2 pinches freshly ground pepper
4 to 6 sprigs fresh parsley, cilantro (coriander), or dill, washed,
     thick stems removed, and minced
¼ cup crumbled blue cheese (optional)
1 to 2 cloves garlic, minced (optional)
1 tablespoon dehydrated onion flakes (optional)
¼ red bell pepper, minced or grated (optional)

1. In a small bowl, mix the yogurt, vinegar or lemon juice, 2 tablespoons water, mustard, sea salt, and pepper. Add the parsley, cilantro, or dill, and stir again.

2. Add any of the optional ingredients, and the 2 additional tablespoons water, if a thinner consistency is preferred.

3. Spoon over a salad, or use as a crudité dip or a sandwich spread.

4. Store leftover dressing in a glass jar in the refrigerator. Shake before using.

Cooking Tip: A versatile food, yogurt creates a creamy dressing that is low in fat and rich in living cultures.

Creamy Balsamic Almond-Butter Dressing

Yield: ¾ cup   100% vegetarian

¼ cup raw almond butter
¼ cup purified water
2 to 3 tablespoons balsamic vinegar
1 tablespoon flaxseed oil or extra-virgin olive oil (optional)
1 clove garlic, peeled and mashed or finely minced
½ teaspoon sea salt

1. In a blender or small bowl, mix the almond butter, water, vinegar, flaxseed oil, if using, garlic, and sea salt.

2. Pour over the salad and toss.

3. Store leftover dressing in a glass jar in the refrigerator. Shake before using.

Cooking Tip: If the oil has separated from the almond paste (or other nut or seed butter), do not throw it out. Use a chopstick or a fork to poke up and down in the paste, allowing the holes to fill with the oil. Eventually it will soften and the oil can be stirred in completely. Place the almond butter in the refrigerator to prevent it from separating again.

 # Chickpea and Red Onion Hummus

Yield: 4½ cups   100% vegetarian

We've devised a fabulous variation of this old standby by using caramelized onions.

PMS Benefits: Chickpeas are a low-fat source of protein. Coupled with a grain, they provide a quality protein equivalent to red meat—a good substitute combination if you find that eating meat worsens menstrual cramping and lower back pain.

4 **tablespoons extra-virgin olive oil**
1 **red onion, chopped**
1 **teaspoon sea salt plus additional as needed**
   Freshly ground pepper
2 **cups cooked chickpeas or other beans (see Note)**
2 **cloves garlic, peeled**
½ **cup lemon juice or ¼ cup cider vinegar and ¼ cup purified water**
2 **tablespoons flaxseed oil**
2 **tablespoons tahini**
   Chickpea cooking liquid or purified water

1. In a medium-sized skillet, on a medium flame, heat 2 tablespoons olive oil and add the onion. Cook until the onion edges begin to turn brown, 7 to 10 minutes. Stir frequently. Sprinkle with a few pinches of sea salt and pepper, stir well, and cook another minute. Set aside.

2. In a blender or food processor, puree the chickpeas, garlic, lemon juice, flaxseed oil, tahini, salt, and the remaining 2 tablespoons olive oil. Puree until smooth, adding ¼ cup amounts of chickpea liquid as needed to allow the machine to blend. The mixture should be smooth and thick.

(Chickpea and Red Onion Hummus—Continued)

3. Using a rubber spatula, scoop the pureed chickpeas into a serving bowl. Top with the cooked and seasoned onion. Serve with Quick Greek Salad (see page 51) and whole-grain pita chips.

Cooking Tip: To use up remaining portions of a dip or spread, use in a sandwich in place of mayonnaise or mustard. Or thin with water (plus a pinch of herbal sea salt) and mix well, pouring this mixture over cooked vegetables, salad greens, grain, pasta, or beans.

Note: Soak 1 cup sorted and washed dried chickpeas in a bowl with 5 cups purified water for 6 hours or overnight. With your hands or a slotted spoon, remove the beans from the water to a saucepan. Add fresh water, and cook according to the bean chart (see page 71). Any of the following cooked beans can be substituted for the chickpeas: navy, Great Northern, cannellini, kidney, adzuki, pinto, or black.

Nutritional Stars: Vitamin C, vitamin E, folic acid, iron, manganese, omega-3 fatty acids

 # The Best Onion-Garlic Dip-o-nnaise

Yield: 2 cups   100% vegetarian

Our tasty "mayonnaise" comes to you without hydrogenated fats, sugar, added chemicals, or extra calories. Spread it on any sandwich, use as a base for salad dressings or dips, or toss a few spoonfuls with seasoned whole-grain pasta.

PMS Benefits: Yogurt made with living bacteria helps to metabolize excess estrogen, thereby lowering the body's estrogen levels and preventing hormonal imbalances. It aids in the breakdown of foods by maintaining a balance of "friendly" bacteria needed for digestion, and also strengthens the immune system. Try yogurt made from whole milk since the fat portion contains all of the essential fat-soluble vitamins such as A, D, E, and K. This kind of yogurt also contains many of the B-complex vitamins and essential fatty acids.

Before you begin, put a colander in a bowl and line it with either paper toweling, coffee filters, or several layers of cheesecloth. Pour in 3 cups plain yogurt with active bacteria (preferably organic) and drain for 2 to 3 hours, refrigerated. This can be done the day before.

 2 **cups drained yogurt (from 3 cups)**
 1 **tablespoon dehydrated onion flakes**
 1 **tablespoon dehydrated garlic flakes or 2 cloves fresh garlic, minced fine**
 2 **tablespoons extra-virgin olive or flaxseed oil**

2 teaspoons dry mustard powder
1 teaspoon cider vinegar or lemon juice
½ to 1 teaspoon herbal sea salt
1 to 2 pinches ground white pepper
2 or 3 sprigs fresh parsley, washed, thick stems removed, and
 minced (optional)
2 to 3 scallions or chives, ends trimmed, and minced (optional)

1. Place the drained yogurt in a medium-sized bowl. Add the onion and garlic flakes and stir well. Add the oil, mustard, vinegar or lemon juice, herbal sea salt, and pepper, and mix thoroughly.

2. Place in the refrigerator for 20 to 30 minutes to moisten the dehydrated vegetables and chill the mixture.

3. Stir in the parsley and chives. Serve with baked corn chips, whole wheat bread sticks, celery and carrot spears, or use as a spread instead of mayonnaise on a sandwich.

Cooking Tip: Look for chemical-free dried onion and garlic flakes. There are now brands prepared from organic vegetables.

Nutritional Stars: Vitamin A, B-complex vitamins, vitamin D

 # Spicy Almond-Butter Spread

Yield: 1½ cups   100% vegetarian

As a spread, serve on bread. For a dip, stir in a little additional water; you can even add more liquid for a sauce that you can drizzle over vegetables, pasta, or grains.

PMS Benefits: Almonds are considered the "queen" of the nuts as they contain many vitamins and minerals. Vitamin B2 aids in the formation of red blood cells; vitamin B3 supports glucose metabolism; vitamin E promotes progesterone production; inositol has a calming effect; calcium prevents cramps and pain; iron prevents anemia; and magnesium helps decrease PMS cramps and control sugar cravings.

½ cup raw almond, tahini, hazelnut, or macadamia butter
½ cup purified water plus additional as needed
2 teaspoons extra-virgin olive oil
1 to 2 teaspoons curry powder
1 clove garlic, peeled and mashed or minced
½ teaspoon sea salt
 Hot sauce (optional)

(Spicy Almond-Butter Spread—Continued)

1. In a medium-sized bowl or blender, mix the nut butter and water until well blended.

2. In a small skillet, heat the oil and cook the curry powder, garlic, and salt briefly. Stir constantly to make sure mixture does not burn. When it begins to bubble, stir once more and immediately add to the nut-butter mixture to stop the cooking.

3. Add a few drops of hot sauce, if desired. Blend well and serve with a fresh vegetable crudité.

Cooking Tip: To mash garlic, flatten the garlic with the broad side of a knife, then chop it with the blade. Add a pinch or two of sea salt and then, again using the side of the knife, mash the garlic back and forth until it has a creamy texture. The salt helps to break down the garlic and preserve its flavor and oils.

Nutritional Stars: B-complex vitamins, vitamin E

Dips and Spreads

Go beyond ordinary chips for dips and spreads!

- **Pita Toast Points:** Slice whole-grain pita bread in half making two disks. Layer them on top of each other and cut into six or eight pieces. Place them in the oven and bake at 350 degrees until golden and crisp. (Or toast whole-grain bread slices cut into quarters.)
- **Vegetable Spears, Medallions, and Slices:** Carrot spears, daikon radish medallions, celery sticks, scallion spears, cucumber rounds or spears, broccoli spears, cauliflower slices, jícama sticks, endive spears, fennel slices, and red, green, and yellow pepper slices.
- **Breads, Crackers, and Chips:** Rye crackers, whole-grain bread cut into quarters, yellow and blue corn chips, whole-grain baguette slices, and sesame whole wheat breadsticks.
- **Corn Tortillas:** Wrap up some dip in a warmed tortilla for a quick and easy meal.

Eat Your Beans

Chili and Other Bean Entrées

The Forgotten Bean: Good Reasons to Include Them in Your Meals

At the turn of the century, Americans ate more legumes (beans, lentils, and peas) than we do today. What a loss, as they meet so many of the requirements of the modern healthy diet. Beans are low in fat and contain only 125 calories per half-cup serving. They are also high in fiber that helps eliminate excess estrogen and ease menstrual woes. Beans are also a valuable source of protein—a half-cup of cooked beans contains the same amount of protein as an ounce and a half of ground beef, about 7 grams. Plus beans supply B vitamins that help a woman manage stress, which can be especially hard to tolerate premenstrually. Finally, beans are high in magnesium, which helps lessen the inflammation associated with breast tenderness. The next time you begin to plan a PMS menu based on a meat entrée, such as pork chops or steak, remind yourself of your nutritional needs and cook up a pot of savory beans instead. (See our section on combining beans with other foods to supply high-quality protein, page 21.)

How to Sort, Wash, Soak, Cook, and Store Beans

1. How to sort beans: Measure the amount of dried beans required by the recipe. Pour the beans into a bowl. Discard stones, cracked beans, and other non-edible items.
2. How to wash beans: Add plenty of purified water to the sorted beans and swish them around with your hand or a spoon. Tilt the bowl and pour most of the water out—just before the beans spill, stop pouring. Depending on the beans, proceed with soaking or cooking. (Refer to the chart on page 71.)
3. How to soak beans: There are two methods for soaking beans.
    A. *Long soaking:* Add plenty of fresh, purified water to the sorted and washed beans (at least 5 cups of water per 1 cup of dried beans). Set the bowl aside, uncovered, for 6 to 8 hours at room temperature. The beans will more than double in size. The beans can also be left to soak overnight or all day while you're away from home.
    B. *Quick soaking:* This is also known as the hot soaking method. After sorting and washing the beans, place them in a saucepan and cover them with 3 to 4 inches of fresh, purified water. Bring the beans to a boil, covered, lower heat, and simmer for 5 minutes. Turn the flame off, and let the beans soak in the hot water for 2 hours, covered.
4. How to cook beans: Using your hands or a slotted spoon, take the beans out of the soaking water and place them in a saucepan. (If the beans were quick-soaked, remove them to a bowl, and rinse the pot to get rid of any dirt that may have settled on the bottom.) Add the desired amount of liquid as called

for in the recipe. Bring the beans to a boil, covered, and proceed with the recipe. Beans are thoroughly cooked when they mash easily when pressed between your fingers or with the tines of a fork.

Other cooking methods include boiling, baking, pressure-cooking, or simmering in a slow cooker. Be forewarned: Never cook green or yellow split peas, or red or green lentils in a pressure cooker, since they tend to foam and clog the cooker's vent.

Do not add salt, sweeteners, fats, tomatoes, or vinegar while beans are cooking since this will harden the skin of the bean and prolong the cooking process. If your beans still haven't softened within the recommended cooking time, they could be old. Try pureeing the semicooked beans and then cooking them for another 10 to 15 minutes. If this alternative method still doesn't soften your beans, discard and start over. If you decide to make a bean salad for lunch, salt your beans after half of the cooking process to keep them from falling apart.

5. How to store beans: Keep glass jars filled with colorful beans labeled for easy identification. Note that you can now purchase tasty cooked beans in jars. Compared to canned beans, jar beans contain no preservatives and less added salt—just in time to treat PMS abdominal bloating!

6. Also see "What to Do with Leftover Cooked Beans," page 22.

Alleviating Gastric Distress

Many people lack the digestive enzyme that breaks down the gas-causing sugars in beans. However, there are ways to cut down on the gas so as to include this healthy food in your meals.

1. Eat beans more frequently.
2. Soak your beans uncovered to reduce digestive gas.
3. Change the soaking water one or two times during the soaking period, allowing the beans to release more gas-producing sugars.
4. Rinse the beans after they have been soaked to remove any remaining sugars.
5. Cook beans in fresh water, not the water they were soaked in.
6. Long-soak the beans rather than quick-soaking them.
7. Reduce or eliminate dairy products in your diet, except for yogurt with living cultures.

To add the missing enzyme: Add a few drops of liquid Beano® to your first bite of beans. This does the trick every time! Call their hotline for a free sample: (800) 257-8650.

Bean Soaking and Cooking Chart

Beans that **Do Not** Need Soaking Before Cooking

Bean type	Cooking time
Adzuki beans[1]	1½ hours
Green lentils	45 minutes
Red lentils	20 minutes
Split peas	1½ hours

[1]Adzuki beans are one of the few beans that do *not* need to be soaked to eliminate the raffinose that produces intestinal gas. But if they are soaked, the cooking time is substantially shortened.

Beans that **Do** Need Soaking Before Cooking

Bean type	Cooking time[1]
Adzuki beans	45 minutes
Anasazi	45 minutes
Black beans	50 minutes
Black-eyed peas	35 minutes
Cannellini beans	60 minutes
Chickpeas	1 to 1½ hours
Great Northern beans	45 minutes
Kidney beans	50 minutes
Lima beans, large	1 hour
Lima beans, small	45 minutes
Navy beans	40 minutes
Pinto beans	45 minutes

[1]When pressure-cooking these beans, reduce the cooking time by half.

Texan Two-step Chili

Yield: 4 to 6 servings   100% vegetarian

A little of this chili and you'll be dancing—but not from the gas of these beans!

PMS Benefits: Beans are very beneficial for PMS relief. A great source of protein, beans are as satisfying and filling as meat, which has a much higher saturated fat content. Women with a lower fat intake tend to have fewer symptoms and more normal levels of estrogen. Beans also contain PMS-fighting zinc, calcium, magnesium, and fiber.

Before you begin, soak 1 cup sorted and washed dried beans, such as pinto, kidney, black, or any white beans, in a bowl with 5 cups purified water for 6 hours or overnight.

    2 cups soaked beans (from 1 cup dried beans)
    5 cups purified water
    4 to 6 tablespoons chili powder
    1 bay leaf
    ¼ cup high-lysine cornmeal or whole-grain bulgur
    3 stalks celery, chopped
    3 cloves garlic, minced
    2 ripe tomatoes, core removed, diced, or one 8-ounce can chopped
          organic tomatoes
    1 or 2 carrots, ends trimmed, chopped
    1 onion, chopped
    1 green bell pepper, seeded and chopped
    1 teaspoon dried oregano
    ¼ cup extra-virgin olive oil or ghee
    2 teaspoons sea salt
       Hot pepper sauce or salsa (optional)
       Hot pepper flakes, cayenne, black or white pepper (optional)
    4 stems fresh cilantro (coriander), thick stems removed, chopped

1. With your hands or a slotted spoon, remove the beans from the soaking water to a saucepan. Add the water, chili powder, and bay leaf. Bring to a boil, covered, reduce flame, and simmer for 30 minutes.

2. Stir the beans and add the cornmeal or bulgur, stirring well. Add the celery, garlic, tomatoes, carrots, onion, bell pepper, and oregano. Stir again, cover, and cook another 20 to 30 minutes. Add additional water if you prefer the chili more liquid.

3. Add the oil or ghee, salt, and, if using, hot pepper sauce and hot pepper flakes. Stir well, taste, and add more seasoning, if desired.

4. Fill large bowls with chili, and top with cilantro. Place a bowl of salsa and one of yogurt on the table for additional garnish. Serve with warm tortillas.

Cooking Tip: For added south-of-the-border flavor, soak dried chili peppers, such as chipotle, jalapeño, serrano, poblano, ancho, mulato, or habarnero. Seed, chop, and add in Step 2.

Variation: For nonvegetarian chili: In a skillet, cook 1 pound chopped meat or small cubes of beef, pork, or chicken in 2 to 3 tablespoons butter until browned. Add to the chili in Step 2.

Nutritional Stars: Calcium, magnesium, zinc

 # Terrine of Blazin' Adzuki Beans and Squash

Yield: 1 loaf   100% vegetarian

We've fused the golden colors of butternut squash with the sweetness of a fresh orange and the rich taste of adzuki beans.

PMS Benefits: The adzuki bean is a small, red Japanese bean laden with zinc and copper. Zinc is important for the growth of female reproductive organs, while copper assists in the development of red blood cells. Insufficient levels of copper can result in anemia and PMS fatigue. The seaweed of this recipe has many PMS-friendly trace minerals.

1 cup dried adzuki beans (will make 2 cups cooked)
4 cups purified water or homemade salt-free vegetarian stock
1 onion, chopped
2 cloves garlic, peeled
1 6-inch strip kelp or kombu seaweed or 1 tablespoon Maine Coast
      seaweed flakes
1 butternut or buttercup squash, ends trimmed, seeded, cut into
      chunks (see Note)
3 slices fresh ginger
½ orange, preferably organic
¼ teaspoon cayenne pepper

(Terrine of Blazin' Adzuki Beans and Squash—Continued)

   3 tablespoons extra-virgin olive oil
   ½ cup whole wheat bread crumbs
   ¼ cup miso paste or 1 teaspoon herbal sea salt
       Pinch ground pepper
   ½ cup raw sunflower seeds

   1. If the adzuki beans have not been soaked, wash them (see page 69). With your hands or a slotted spoon, remove the beans from the washing water and place them in a medium-sized saucepan with the fresh water or stock, onion, garlic, and kelp or kombu. Bring to a boil, covered, lower flame, and simmer for 30 minutes.

   2. Add the squash, ginger, orange, and cayenne. Return to a boil, covered, reduce flame, and simmer until the beans are soft, another 30 to 50 minutes (depending on whether or not the beans were soaked).

   3. Adjust the oven shelves to fit a loaf pan. Preheat the oven to 350 degrees.

   4. Place a colander in a bowl, and pour the beans in to drain. (Save the cooking liquid for a soup or use as a stock.)

   5. In a food processor, puree the drained bean mixture until smooth. Add the oil, ¼ cup bread crumbs, miso paste or herbal sea salt, and pepper. Puree again until well blended and smooth.

   6. Prepare a loaf pan by oiling the bottom and sides. Add the remaining ¼ cup bread crumbs and shake the pan to distribute evenly. Using a rubber spatula or spoon, scrape the bean mixture into the loaf pan. Smooth the top with the spatula or back of spoon. (You may also use a flat baking casserole for the bean mixture, which can later be cut into squares.) Top with the sunflower seeds, pressing them lightly into the beans.

   7. Put the bean loaf in the oven and cook for 40 to 50 minutes. The top will brown slightly and the edges begin to pull away from the sides of the pan.

   8. Remove the loaf from the oven and cool for 10 to 15 minutes.

   9. To remove the bean loaf from the pan, slide a paring knife around the perimeter of the pan, loosening the loaf. Place a cutting board or large platter on top of the loaf pan and, holding both at the same time, invert the loaf and board. Carefully lift the loaf pan off; the loaf is now ready to be sliced.

   Cooking Tip: Though adzuki beans require no soaking, a standard 6- to 8-hour or overnight soaking will reduce the cooking time by 30 minutes.

   Note: If the skin of the squash is waxed, please peel it.

   Nutritional Stars: Folic acid, copper, zinc

Black Bean Timbales with Pumpkinseeds

Yield: 8 to 12 timbales   100% vegetarian

This dish tops a hearty mix of pureed beans with zinc-rich pumpkinseeds, good for women—and men too! Our timbales are easy to reheat or to use in sandwiches.

PMS Benefits: A rich source of vitamin B2, copper, iron, magnesium, and zinc, pumpkinseeds help treat a woman with PMS symptoms.

Before you begin, soak 1 cup sorted and washed dried black beans (or other favorite beans) in a bowl with 5 cups purified water for 6 hours or overnight.

2 **cups soaked black beans (from 1 cup dried beans)**
4 **cups purified water or homemade salt-free vegetarian stock**
1 **onion, quartered**
2 **cloves garlic, peeled**
1 **bay leaf**
3 **tablespoons extra-virgin olive oil**
½ **cup whole-grain bread crumbs**
¼ **cup miso paste or 1 teaspoon herbal sea salt**
2 **tablespoons mustard**
¼ **teaspoon ground pepper**
2 **teaspoons dried savory**
1 **teaspoon dried tarragon**
½ **cup raw, shelled pumpkinseeds**

1. With your hands or a slotted spoon, remove the beans from the soaking water and put them in a medium-sized saucepan with the fresh water or stock, onion, garlic, and bay leaf. Bring to a boil, covered, lower flame, and simmer until the beans are soft, about 50 minutes.

2. Adjust the oven shelves to fit a loaf pan. Preheat the oven to 350 degrees.

3. Place a colander in a bowl, and pour in the beans. Discard the bay leaf. Put the drained beans and vegetables in a food processor and puree until smooth. Add the oil, ¼ cup bread crumbs, miso paste or herbal sea salt, mustard, pepper, and herbs. Puree again until well blended and smooth.

4. Prepare a muffin tin by oiling each of the cups on the bottom and sides. Add the remaining ¼ cup bread crumbs to the cups and shake the pan to distribute evenly. Using a large spoon, fill each muffin cup with the bean mixture. Smooth the

(Black Bean Timbales with Pumpkinseeds—Continued)

top with the back of the spoon. Top each timbale with pumpkinseeds. Press them slightly into the top of the bean mixture.

5. Put the muffin pan in the oven and cook for 25 to 35 minutes. The tops will brown slightly, the edges will begin to pull away from the sides of the pan, and the pumpkinseeds will turn slightly golden.

6. Remove from the oven and cool for 5 to 10 minutes.

7. To remove the timbales from the muffin cups, loosen the timbales by sliding a paring knife around the perimeter of each muffin cup. Place a cutting board or large platter on top of the muffin pan and, holding both at the same time, invert the muffin pan and the board. Lift off the muffin pan. Serve two or three timbales per person. The timbales are now ready to be eaten—add some salsa and cilantro.

Cooking Tip: Use a pastry brush to speed the oiling of the muffin-pan cups or fill them with paper muffin cups and omit the oiling.

Nutritional Stars: Vitamin B2, copper, iron, magnesium, zinc

 # Caribbean Twice-cooked Pinto Beans with Plantains

Yield: 6 servings   100% vegetarian

Steel drums, warm air, clean beaches, and soul-satisfying food. Bring home a piece of the Caribbean while feeding your family and friends a satisfying and nurturing meal.

PMS Benefits: Plantains contain vitamin B6, which helps form serotonin, the brain chemical that calms your mood. They are also rich in magnesium, which is important for brain, nerve, and muscle cells to function properly.

Before you begin, soak 1 cup sorted and washed dried pinto beans (or other favorite beans) in a bowl with 5 cups purified water for 6 hours or overnight.

2 **cups soaked pinto beans (from 1 cup dried beans)**
6 **cups purified water or homemade salt-free vegetable stock**
4 **cloves garlic, minced**
1 **carrot, ends trimmed, chopped**
2 **tablespoons unsulphured blackstrap molasses**
1 **bay leaf**
6 **tablespoons unsalted butter, preferably organic, or ghee (see page 227)**

2 **tablespoons chili or curry powder**
2 **red onions, sliced**
2 **yellow onions, sliced**
1 **ripe plantain**
   Grated zest of 1 orange, preferably organic
1 **teaspoon powdered ginger**
½ **to 1 teaspoon sea salt**
½ **teaspoon nutmeg**
½ **teaspoon ground pepper**
½ **cup unsweetened apple juice**

1. With your hands or a slotted spoon, remove the beans from the soaking water and put in a saucepan with the fresh water or stock, garlic, carrot, molasses, and bay leaf. Bring to a boil, covered, lower flame, and simmer until the beans are soft, about 45 minutes.

2. In a medium-sized skillet, heat 2 tablespoons butter or ghee. Add the chili or curry powder, stir briefly, and add the onions. Cook on medium-high heat, uncovered, stirring occasionally until brown and caramelized, 10 to 15 minutes. Remove to a bowl.

3. Peel the plantain, and cut into ½-inch rounds. Set aside.

4. In the same skillet in which the onions were cooked (without rinsing the skillet), melt 2 tablespoons butter or ghee on medium heat. Add the orange zest, ginger, sea salt, nutmeg, and black pepper. Stir briefly and cook just until the spices bubble. Add the plantains and apple juice. Lower heat to a simmer, cover, and cook for 5 minutes. Remove from flame and set aside.

5. Heat a large skillet, and melt the remaining 2 tablespoons butter or ghee on medium heat. With a slotted spoon, take the beans and vegetables from the cooking liquid and put in the skillet. Add enough cooking liquid to cover the beans halfway, and cook on a medium-high flame, uncovered. Using a wooden spoon, occasionally stir and mash the beans and vegetables against the side of the skillet. Add more cooking liquid as the beans thicken and become like a paste. This process takes 15 to 20 minutes. If you prefer a looser bean paste, after adding the remaining liquid, stir and remove from the stove.

6. Add the caramelized onions and the spiced plantains. Stir and cook another 3 or 4 minutes.

Cooking Tip: The plantain is a type of banana that is used in much of the southern hemisphere. It can be eaten in every stage of development—when the peel is green to yellow, the flesh is bland and starchy and can be used like the white potato. As the peel changes to yellow-brown, and even becomes black, the plantain can be used both as a fruit and a vegetable—the flesh is now sweet and has a banana aroma. When cooked, the plantain maintains its shape, at all stages.

Nutritional Stars: Vitamin B6, B-complex vitamins, magnesium

South African Navy Bean Croquette Logs

Yield: 4 servings   100% vegetarian

These nutrient-rich logs make great traveling food—but they are also ideal for supper. Add soup and a salad to complete your PMS meal.

PMS Benefits: Antioxidants are important to protect the body from free-radical damage that can occur when you are exposed to environmental pollutants such as smog and secondhand cigarette smoke. Vitamin E is one of the most important of the antioxidants, especially when coupled with vitamins A and C, and the mineral selenium. Navy beans are a good source of this very needed vitamin.

Before you begin, soak 1 cup sorted and washed dried navy beans in a bowl with 5 cups purified water for 6 hours or overnight.

- 2 **cups soaked navy beans (from 1 cup dried beans)**
- 5 **cups purified water or homemade salt-free vegetable stock**
- 2 **teaspoons turmeric powder**
- 1 **bay leaf**
- ½ **lemon with rind, preferably organic**
- ½ **cinnamon stick**
- 2 **cloves garlic, peeled and quartered**
- 1 **onion, quartered**
- ½ **bunch fresh cilantro (coriander), washed, thick stems removed, and minced**
- 1 **teaspoon herbal sea salt**
- 1 **tablespoon prepared mustard**
- ¼ to ½ **cup bread crumbs**
- ½ **cup unsulphured currants**
- ½ **cup high-lysine cornmeal**
- ¼ to ½ **cup ghee, preferably organic (see page 227)**
- ¼ to ½ **cup extra-virgin olive oil**

1. With your hands or a slotted spoon, remove the beans from the soaking water and place in a saucepan with the fresh water or stock, turmeric, bay leaf, lemon, and cinnamon stick. Bring to a boil, covered, lower flame, and simmer until the beans are soft, about 50 minutes.

2. Place a colander in a bowl. Pour in the beans and liquid and drain well. (Use the cooking liquid for soup or save for stock.) Remove the bay leaf, lemon, and cinnamon stick, and discard.

3. In a blender or food processor, pulse-mince the garlic, onion, and cilantro. Add the beans and herbal sea salt. (Or mince the vegetables fine by hand and, using a potato masher, pulverize the beans. Stir together and proceed.) Add the mustard and ¼ cup bread crumbs to bind the mixture. Stir again. Add the currants and more bread crumbs, if needed.

4. Put the cornmeal in a wide bowl or plate. Wet your hands lightly and form 1 × 3-inch logs (or 3 × ½-inch patties) with the bean mixture. (Make sure the ends are blunt and not tapered.) Place the logs in the cornmeal and roll to cover them completely; remove to a plate until all the logs have been made.

5. In a large skillet, heat ¼ cup ghee and ¼ cup olive oil. Cook the logs until golden. Use two forks to turn the logs until all sides have browned. Remove to a brown bag or paper toweling.

6. Serve with hot sauce, a side of salsa or lemon wedges, a hearty raw salad, and a loaf of bread for a complete protein.

Cooking Tip: As the main ingredient of curry powder, turmeric gives curry its yellow color. You can use curry powder as a substitute if you do not have plain turmeric.

Note: Any favorite bean can be substituted for the navy beans, such as anasazi, black, kidney, pinto, chickpea, or black-eyed peas.

Nutritional Stars: Vitamin A, vitamin C, magnesium, selenium

 # Lima Beans, Corn, and Green Bean Succotash

Yield: 4 to 6 servings   100% vegetarian

We love this classic American combination of creamy lima beans, crunchy corn, and green beans. Transform leftover succotash into a delicious soup by adding some homemade stock. Succotash is even good spread on toast.

PMS Benefits: All white beans, such as lima beans, have appreciable amounts of calcium and magnesium. Limas also contain vitamin B6 and iron, among the most important nutrients for a woman with PMS, as they help to steady nerves and ease cramps.

(Lima Beans, Corn, and Green Bean Succotash—Continued)

Before you begin, soak 1 cup sorted and washed dried lima beans in a bowl with 5 cups purified water for 6 hours or overnight.

   2 **cups soaked lima beans (from 1 cup dried beans)**
   4 **cups purified water or homemade salt-free vegetable stock**
   2 **tablespoons unsalted butter, preferably organic**
   1 **onion, chopped**
     Kernels from 2 ears fresh corn
 ¼ **pound green beans, tips removed, cut in half**
 ½ **teaspoon sea salt**
 ⅛ **teaspoon paprika**
   3 **to 4 sprigs fresh parsley, washed, thick stems removed, and minced**

1. With your hands or a slotted spoon, remove the beans from the soaking water and put in a saucepan with the fresh water or stock. Bring to a boil, covered, lower flame, and simmer until the beans are soft, about 50 minutes.

2. In a large sauté pan, melt the butter and add the onion. Cook on medium heat, covered, until the onion is translucent, about 10 minutes. Add the cooked beans with half the cooking liquid, the corn kernels, green beans, sea salt, and paprika. Cover and bring to a boil. Reduce heat, leave lid partially uncovered, and cook until the corn and beans are tender, about 15 minutes. Stir occasionally. Add more bean liquid if the mixture begins to dry out.

3. Stir in the parsley, and cook uncovered for another 2 or 3 minutes.

Cooking Tip: To remove the kernels from the corn, first shuck or remove the outer husk. Break the cob in half, and set the broken end down on a cutting board with the cob sticking straight up. Carefully hold the cob and, with your fingers out of the way, slide a chef's knife down the kernels, slicing them off. Turn the cob, and continue until all have been removed. Continue with the other pieces. Once the kernels have been removed, the leftover cobs make a sweet-tasting stock.

Nutritional Stars: Vitamin B6, calcium, magnesium, iron

Braised Tofu with Fennel in Parsley Cream Sauce

Yield: 4 servings   100% vegetarian

Here is a satisfying dish that combines the smooth texture of tofu with the slight crunch of fennel. The overall flavor is one of fresh herbs. We finish it by adding a splash of cream to give the dish a hint of richness. There are many ways to flavor tofu beyond using soy sauce!

PMS Benefits: Soy foods can help balance hormones and lessen symptoms of PMS, as they contain high levels of especially potent phytohormones called isoflavones. These are also present in chickpeas.

3 **tablespoons unsalted butter, preferably organic**
1½ **pounds firm tofu, diced**
1 **bulb fresh fennel**
2 **tablespoons extra-virgin olive oil**
1 **onion, sliced thin**
8 to 10 **button mushrooms, washed and cut in half**
3 **sprigs fresh parsley, washed, thick stems removed, minced**
2 **tablespoons cream, preferably organic**
½ **teaspoon sea salt**
¼ **teaspoon ground pepper**

1. In a large skillet over high heat, melt 2 tablespoons butter. Add the tofu and cook until golden brown, about 10 minutes, turning frequently with a metal spatula. Remove to a plate and set aside.

2. Remove the top stalks from the fennel and trim the end. Cut the bulb in half vertically. Remove the core and discard. Cut the fennel halves into thin slices.

3. To the same skillet, add the remaining 1 tablespoon butter with the olive oil. Add the onion and cook on medium heat, uncovered, until it begins to soften, about 5 minutes. Stir occasionally.

4. Add the mushrooms, fennel, and parsley, and stir. Continue to cook until the vegetables are tender, about 10 minutes. Stir occasionally.

5. Lower heat, and stir in the tofu, cream, salt, and pepper. Cook another 2 minutes, stirring occasionally.

6. Serve immediately with slices of crusty whole-grain bread and vegetable soup.

Cooking Tip: A small amount of cream and/or butter added to a recipe imparts a luxurious amount of flavor.

Nutritional Stars: B-complex vitamins, calcium, potassium

The Whole-Grain and Pasta Story

Whole Grains

Whole-Grain Pastas

Why Whole Grains Are So Important

Fight your PMS with whole grains, an excellent source of all the major nutrient groups—carbohydrates, protein, fats, vitamins, and minerals. Whole grains are a great source of the B vitamins, minerals such as magnesium, plus insoluble fiber, which helps to remove estrogen from the body. This helps balance hormonal levels and prevent menstrual symptoms such as anxiety.

Like beans, grains are not a complete protein because they lack some of the amino acids that are essential for health. When you eat grain as your protein source remember to combine it with foods that can supply the missing protein, ingredients such as beans, nuts, seeds, seafood, and poultry. Vegetarians in particular who are not careful about proper protein intake can develop a protein deficiency, signs of which include cravings for sweets—especially in full-time vegetarians. And satisfying this hunger with sugary sweets can only increase your symptoms of PMS.

When you are combining grains and beans, mix $1\frac{1}{2}$ to 2 parts whole grains to 1 part beans, or $\frac{3}{4}$ to 1 cup of grains to $\frac{1}{2}$ cup of beans. If you substitute seeds or nuts for beans, 2 tablespoons of these to 1 cup of grain is sufficient.

How to Wash, Drain, Cook, and Store Grains

Whole grains that have not been through the refining process will contain dust and chaff. Before cooking these grains, you'll need to wash them thoroughly; we'll teach you our method for really cleaning away the dirt!

1. How to wash whole grains: Measure the amount of grain required by the recipe (usually 1 cup) and pour it into a medium-sized saucepan. Cover the grain with at least 3 to 4 inches of purified water. Using your hand or a spoon, swish the grain around to loosen any dust and inedible fibers. These will float to the top.
   A. *Wash these grains:* Rice (brown, wehani, basmati, wild, and Arborio), barley, millet, quinoa, whole wheat, rye, and any other whole grain.
   B. *Do not wash these grains:* Pasta, kasha, bulgur, couscous, and any grain that has been cut, flaked, broken, or rolled, such as steel-cut and rolled oats.
2. How to drain whole grains: Have a medium- or fine-meshed sieve available, large enough to hold all of the measured grain (the holes of a colander are too large). Tilt the saucepan, pouring out as much of the water as possible into the sink, then pour the remaining grain and water into the sieve. Return the grain to the saucepan. (If the washing water is very dirty, repeat this cleaning process.)
3. How to cook whole grains: We usually use water for cooking grain, but if you prefer added flavor, choose a favorite stock. Measure the amount of liquid

required by the recipe and proceed with the cooking instructions. Bring the grain, liquid, and salt to a boil in a covered saucepan. Lower the flame and cook the specified amount of time. If the saucepan is thin-bottomed or you are cooking on an electric stove, place a heat diffuser between the flame and the pot. The heat will steam the grain, which should remain unstirred for the total cooking period. Turn off the heat and allow the grain to sit covered for 5 to 10 minutes, time permitting. (Cook individual grains according to the recipe instructions, or see the chart below.)

4. How to store whole grains: We prefer to store our grains in glass jars, with a stick-on label for easy identification. To keep moths from hatching in the jar and infesting your grain, add a bay leaf.

Whole-Grain Pasta

We've found many whole-grain pastas on the market that taste great, and we frequently interchange these pastas with recipes that call for white-flour or semolina pasta. See pages 94–95 for more information.

Whole-Grain Cooking Chart		
Whole grain[1]	**Liquid**	**Cooking time**
Arborio rice	3 to 4 cups	1 hour
Barley, slightly pearled	2 cups	1 hour
Brown rice, long grain	1½ cups	55 minutes
Brown rice, short grain	2 cups	55 minutes
Bulgur[2]	1½ cups, boiling	10 minutes
Cornmeal, high-lysine[2]	4 to 5 cups	45 minutes
Couscous, whole grain[2]	1½ cups, boiling	10 minutes
Kasha (buckwheat)[2]	2 cups, boiling	10 minutes
Millet	2 cups	35 minutes
Oatmeal, rolled[2]	2 cups	20 minutes
Oats, steel-cut[2]	2 cups	30 minutes
Pasta, whole grain[2]	2 quarts	7 to 10 minutes
Quinoa	2 cups	15 minutes
Soba[2]	2 quarts	7 to 10 minutes
Udon[2]	2 quarts	7 to 10 minutes
Wild rice	3 cups	1 hour

[1] 1 cup grain or 8 ounces pasta.

[2] Requires no washing.

Vegetable Paella Primer

Yield: 6 servings   100% vegetarian

Paella is a terrific crowd-pleasing, all-in-one-meal dish. Feel free to design the paella according to your own palette, and choose from a wonderful assortment of seasonal vegetables. To turn this paella into the traditional nonvegetarian and Spanish classic, add seafood and chicken pieces.

PMS Benefits: High-fat and low-fiber diets put a woman at risk for elevated estrogen levels that trigger uncomfortable PMS symptoms. The whole grains and vegetables we use in this recipe contain the fiber your body uses to treat its PMS. There's also a bonus in using brown rice, which contains 172 mg of magnesium per cup versus 13 mg per cup in white rice. Magnesium eases menstrual cramps and stabilizes emotions.

2 **cups brown rice, washed (see page 85 and Note 1)**
¼ **teaspoon saffron**
5 **cups homemade salt-free vegetable stock or purified water**
1½ **teaspoons sea salt plus additional if needed**
4 **tablespoons unsalted butter, preferably organic**
2 **onions, chopped**
3 **to 4 cloves garlic, minced**
2 **stalks broccoli, stalks peeled, cut into bite-sized pieces**
1 **small head cauliflower, core removed, cut into bite-sized pieces**
2 **stalks celery, ends trimmed, chopped**
2 **to 3 ripe tomatoes, cores removed, chopped**
2 **carrots, ends trimmed, chopped**
1 **red bell pepper, seeded and chopped**
¼ **teaspoon ground pepper**

1. In a large saucepan, bring the washed rice, saffron, 4 cups stock or water, and 1½ teaspoons salt to a boil, covered. Lower flame and simmer for 50 minutes.

2. In a large skillet or chef's pan, melt the butter and add the onions and garlic. Sauté until they begin to brown at the edges, about 10 minutes.

3. Add the broccoli, cauliflower, celery, tomatoes, carrots, red pepper, and the remaining 1 cup stock or water. Cover and bring to a boil. Lower flame and cook 5 to 7 minutes. (See Note 2. For nonvegetarian paella, add the clams, lobster, mussels, chicken, shrimp, fish fillet, scallops, or additional vegetables at this point and cook thoroughly.)

(Vegetable Paella Primer—Continued)

4. Add the cooked rice, and season with salt and pepper to taste. Serve in large bowls with a salad on the side.

Cooking Tip: Saffron is the yellow-orange stigma of a small purple crocus. The stigmas are handpicked and dried—it takes over 14,000 stigmas for each ounce of saffron. The spices turmeric and annatto are used as substitutes for the color of saffron, but do not duplicate its unique pungent and aromatic flavor.

Note 1: Rice is the most familiar paella grain, though we tempt you to experiment with the delicious consistency of barley, quinoa, or millet.

Note 2: Add all of the following or any that you prefer: 8 clams, 1 lobster (cut into 8 to 10 pieces), 10 mussels, ½ chicken (cut into 8 pieces), 12 shrimp, 1 fish fillet, or 8 scallops, and any additional vegetables.

Nutritional Stars: B-complex vitamins, iron, manganese, zinc

 ## Rice 'n Barley and Asparagus Risotto

Yield: 4 servings   100% vegetarian

We've prepared an enticing new way to eat asparagus. The soft and creamy texture of barley and rice envelop the stalks, while the bright green spears add color and a slight crunch to your meal.

PMS Benefits: Vegetables, dried peas and beans, and whole grains contain complex carbohydrates, which supply fiber and starch. Such foods steady blood sugar and moods.

½ **cup brown rice, washed (see page 85 and Cooking Tip)**
½ **cup barley, washed**
  Large pinch saffron
3 **cups homemade salt-free vegetable stock or purified water**
1 **bunch asparagus (1 to 1½ pounds), tough ends removed**
2 **tablespoons unsalted butter, preferably organic, or extra-virgin olive oil**
1 **teaspoon herbal sea salt**
½ **teaspoon ground white pepper**

1. In a large saucepan, put the rice and barley, saffron, and 1½ cups stock or water. Bring to a boil and cook, uncovered, on a medium flame. Stir frequently.

2. In a medium-sized saucepan, warm the remaining stock, covered. It is not necessary for it to come to a boil.

3. As the rice cooks and the liquid is absorbed, stir in additional stock, ½ cup at a time. Stir well after each addition. Continue this process until all of the stock has been used. The kernels of grain will be soft, and yet chewy and creamy.

4. Break the asparagus tips off and set aside. Slice the stems into thin rounds. Stir in the asparagus stems, butter or olive oil, herbal sea salt, and pepper. Cook for 1 minute. Add the tips and stir again, cooking for another 1 or 2 minutes, uncovered. (Additional liquid can be added, if needed.) Serve hot, along with beans, poultry, or meat with a salad.

Cooking Tip: You'll find many varieties of brown rice in your local natural-food store. Long, short, and medium-grain brown rices are the most common, but now Arborio rice—the typical risotto grain—is also available in the whole-grain form.

Nutritional Stars: B-complex vitamins, boron, potassium

About Barley

Pearled barley, which is commonly sold in the grocery store, is a small, round grain, the result of the refining process. Better-quality barley is one that has some of its bran and germ intact. It has an almost oval shape and is tan or light brown, and has been only slightly refined. Look for this nutritious grain in your natural-food store, where it is also called pearl barley. Whole barley, also found in specialty stores, is truly oval and dark brown, and is what pearled barley is made from. It requires 4 to 6 hours of soaking before cooking. We've developed our PMS-banishing recipes using the slightly pearled variety of barley.

 # Millet-stuffed Collards Baked with Apricots and Prunes

Yield: 8 to 12 collard rolls   100% vegetarian

These collards are just as good stuffed with kasha or bulgur instead of the millet. All three grains cook quickly and they are all good for PMS.

PMS Benefits: Many foods contain fiber, an important element for both maintaining a woman's overall health and treating PMS symptoms. Fiber helps to remove toxins from the system. You'll find fiber in the millet, fresh collards, apricots, and prunes.

(Millet-stuffed Collards Baked with Apricots and Prunes—Continued)

3½ **cups homemade salt-free vegetable stock or purified water**
1 **cup millet, washed (see page 85)**
2 **mint tea bags or 2 sprigs fresh mint, leaves only, minced**
2 **tablespoons unsalted butter, preferably organic**
1 **teaspoon herbal sea salt**
2 **quarts purified water**
1 **bunch collards, at least 8 leaves**
2 **cloves garlic, minced**
1 **onion, minced**
2 **tablespoons extra-virgin olive oil**
  Grated zest of 1 lemon, preferably organic
¼ **teaspoon ground pepper**
½ **cup unsulphured dried apricots**
½ **cup unsulphured dried prunes, pitted**
1 **recipe Creamy Mushroom Sauce with Golden Garlic Bits**
  (see page 201) or Sweet Red Pepper Butter (see page 202)
2 **or 3 sprigs fresh parsley or additional mint, washed**

1. In a medium-sized saucepan, put 2 cups stock or water, the millet, mint, butter, and herbal sea salt. Bring to a boil, covered. Lower flame and cook 30 minutes.

2. In a large pot, bring 2 quarts water to a boil, covered. Meanwhile, remove the collard stems at the base of the leaf. Using a paring knife, thin the rib by cutting a sliver of the thick rib off each leaf. (This will allow it more flexibility.) Drop the leaves into the boiling water and cook uncovered for 5 minutes.

3. Place a colander in the sink and drain the collards, discarding the water. Set aside to cool.

4. Discard the tea bags, if used. With a fork, scratch the surface of the millet to fluff and separate grains. Scoop the millet into a large bowl. Add the garlic, onion, olive oil, lemon zest, and pepper. Stir well to mix and let cool. Once cool enough to touch, using your hands, mash the millet to form a sticky stuffing.

5. Position the oven shelves so that a medium-sized baking pan will fit in the center. Preheat the oven to 350 degrees.

6. Cover the bottom of the baking pan with the apricots and prunes. Add 1½ cups stock or water.

7. On a large work surface, lay out several collard leaves. Put a large spoonful of the filling in the center of a leaf, 1 or 2 inches from the cut stem end. Begin by covering the filling with one end of the collard leaf, then fold the sides over each other. Finish the rolling by completely enclosing the interior. Place the collard roll, seam side down, in the baking pan on top of the dried fruit, laying the rolls next to each other. Continue until all of the collards or the filling have been used up.

8. Cover with parchment paper and foil, and bake in the preheated oven for 40 to 45 minutes.

9. In a small saucepan, warm up the sauce you have chosen. Carefully place the collards on a deep serving platter. Spoon the apricots and prunes along the outer rim of the platter. Garnish with the parsley. Put the sauce in a gravy boat with a ladle, and serve it on the side.

Cooking Tip: Many cooks dry-roast millet to give it more flavor. Instead of adding another step, we added a small amount of butter, which brightens the taste.

Nutritional Stars: B complex, vitamin E, boron, iron

 # Bulgur Pilaf with Cremini Mushrooms and Roasted Sunflower Seeds

Yield: 4 servings   100% vegetarian

All versions of pilaf have always been favorites with our families and friends. Here we make it with one of the quickest-cooking grains imaginable and bring to you its whole-grain nutrition.

PMS Benefits: The B vitamins, including vitamin B6, need to be consumed in their natural proportions, such as that found in whole grains. An imbalance will disturb the intestinal flora and cause some vitamins to be excreted. Whole wheat contains vitamins B1, B2, B3, B6, folic acid, and inositol, as well as vitamin E and the minerals calcium, iron, magnesium, and zinc. Its refined cousin doesn't compare.

- 2 **tablespoons unsalted butter, preferably organic**
- 4 **ounces cremini mushrooms or button mushrooms, washed and sliced**
- 2 **cloves garlic, minced**
- ½ **teaspoon dried thyme**
   Herbal sea salt
- ¼ **teaspoon ground pepper**
- 2 **cups homemade salt-free vegetable stock or purified water**
- 1 **cup whole-grain bulgur**
- ½ **cup raw sunflower or pumpkinseeds**
- ½ **teaspoon chili powder**
- ¼ **teaspoon garlic powder**

(Bulgur Pilaf with Cremini Mushrooms and Roasted Sunflower Seeds—Continued)

1. In a medium-sized sauté pan, heat the butter and add the mushrooms, garlic, thyme, 1 teaspoon herbal sea salt, and pepper. Cook on moderate heat, covered, until the mushrooms release their juices, 5 to 7 minutes.

2. In a medium-sized saucepan, bring the stock or water to a boil, covered. Add the bulgur, cover, lower flame, and simmer for 10 minutes. Remove from heat and set aside for 10 minutes.

3. In a small skillet, dry-roast the sunflower seeds or pumpkinseeds with the chili and garlic powders, and a pinch of herbal sea salt. Stir constantly to prevent burning. The seeds will begin to pop and smell toasted. As soon as they are cooked, remove to a plate to cool. (Do not leave them in the skillet or they will burn.)

4. Using a fork, scratch the surface of the cooked bulgur to fluff and separate grains. Spoon into a serving bowl. Top with the roasted sunflower seeds or pumpkinseeds and serve hot.

Cooking Tip: Bulgur is available made either from whole wheat or refined wheat. We recommend you cook with the slightly darker whole wheat bulgur, available in the bulk bins of your local natural-food store. Packaged bulgur or the kind sold in Middle Eastern stores is made from polished wheat, which lacks the valuable bran and germ.

Nutritional Stars: B-complex vitamins, inositol, vitamin E, calcium, iron, magnesium, zinc

Polenta Cups with Chunky Onion-Celery Tomato Sauce

Yield: 4 servings   100% vegetarian

When hot, polenta will take the shape of any mold. Here we pour our polenta into a muffin pan to make individual servings. After ladling a generous helping of sauce onto your plate, top it with several polenta domes!

PMS Benefits: Calcium and magnesium help to prevent PMS cramping and pain. Cornmeal contains both of these minerals.

   5   **cups purified water**
1½   **cups high-lysine cornmeal**
   1   **teaspoon herbal sea salt**
   3   **tablespoons unsalted butter, preferably organic, or extra-virgin olive oil**

½ **teaspoon ground white pepper**
1 **recipe Chunky Onion-Celery Tomato Sauce (see page 203)**
   Grated cheese (optional)

1. Put the water into a medium-sized saucepan and whisk in the cornmeal and herbal sea salt. Bring to a boil, stirring frequently to prevent the cornmeal from settling on the bottom of the pot. At first use the whisk, and as the cornmeal thickens, change to a wooden spoon.

2. Reduce heat, cover, and simmer for 35 minutes. (If you are cooking on an electric stove or have a thin-bottomed pot, put a heat diffuser between the heating element and the saucepan.) Stir occasionally. The cornmeal will be thick; if needed, stir in a small amount of additional water.

3. Turn off flame and add the butter and pepper. Cover for a few minutes to allow the butter to melt, then stir it in.

4. Fit the muffin pan with paper liners or rinse the insides of the cups with cold water, leaving them wet. Spoon the cornmeal into each cup, filling it to the top. Set aside to cool and solidify, 15 to 20 minutes.

5. In a saucepan, heat the Chunky Onion-Celery Tomato Sauce. Spread a thick layer of the sauce on a serving platter. Unmold the polenta cups and remove the paper liners, if used, and place them on the sauce top side down. Serve the extra sauce in a gravy boat on the side with grated cheese, if desired.

Cooking Tip: To prevent cornmeal from lumping as it begins to cook, it should always be added to cold or room-temperature water. An alternative to preparing cornmeal from scratch is to buy the ready-made variety, which comes in thick, sausage-shaped tubes. Cut each tube into round slices and sauté in butter to make a tasty side dish, or unwrap a tube of polenta, soften it by adding a little water and by heating the polenta, and use as this recipe suggests.

Nutritional Stars: Vitamin C, calcium, magnesium

 # Millet Pilaf with Vermicelli Noodles

Yield: 4 servings   100% vegetarian

Based on traditional rice pilaf with egg noodles, this satisfying whole-grain dish will bring smiles to all those who share it with you.

PMS Benefits: Complex carbohydrates require a lot more of time to break down compared with refined sugar, since starch molecules are much larger than sucrose

(Millet Pilaf with Vermicelli Noodles—Continued)

and complex carbohydrates also contain a small amount of fat and protein. This process has a gentler effect on your blood sugar, holding it steady as well as keeping your PMS mood swings at bay.

> 1 **cup millet, washed (see page 85)**
> ¼ **cup unsalted butter, preferably organic, or extra-virgin olive oil**
> ½ **cup whole wheat vermicelli noodles or broken whole-grain pasta**
> 2½ **cups homemade salt-free vegetable stock or purified water**
> 1 **teaspoon herbal sea salt**
> ½ **cup fresh corn kernels (1 ear of corn) or ½ cup fresh peas (optional)**

1. Pour the washed millet into a fine-meshed sieve and drain well.

2. In a medium-sized saucepan, on moderate heat, melt the butter or oil. Add the millet and toast, stirring frequently, until it begins to brown and smell toasted. Add the noodles and cook another 2 to 3 minutes, continuing to stir. Be careful not to burn.

3. Carefully, add the stock or water in ½-cup amounts until 1½ cups have been added. Pour in the rest of the liquid and the herbal sea salt. Stir once, cover, and bring to a boil. Lower the flame and simmer for 20 minutes.

4. Add the corn or peas, if using, to the top of the cooking millet. Do not stir. Cover and continue cooking for 10 more minutes.

5. Using a fork, scratch the surface of the millet to fluff and separate grains, stirring the corn in. Spoon into a serving bowl and serve hot.

Cooking Tip: Save time and trouble by making this pilaf without roasting the grain. You'll notice the difference in taste, though, as roasted grains have a richer and nuttier feel. In this recipe, we suggest using stock instead of water as the cooking liquid, a substitution which adds its own richness.

Nutritional Stars: B-complex vitamins, boron, iron, magnesium

Pasta Basics

Ahhhh! The virtues of pasta . . . Pasta continues to be known for being low fat and quick cooking, and for being a dish almost anyone will enjoy.

Here's the catch—most pasta is made from semolina flour, which is the refined variety of durum wheat. It has been stripped of over twenty-two nutrients, including its fiber, and then enriched with three or four nutrients. This can hardly be called a nutritious food! And don't be fooled by spinach or artichoke pastas—these are refined white-flour versions with a little vegetable added for color.

Whole-grain pasta is readily available in the natural-food store. The Japanese have made it for centuries. There is soba made from buckwheat flour, and udon that is made with whole wheat flour. And there are now many whole wheat pasta shapes on the market—vermicelli, fettuccini, spirals, ribbons, lasagna, elbows, spaghetti, angel hair, and shells. If you are sensitive to wheat, look for corn, rice, spelt, quinoa, and kamut pastas. In addition, couscous, a Mideastern pasta, is now available in its whole-grain form. It still has a 10-minute cooking time and contains all its natural nutrients and fiber.

The whole-grain pastas still offer all the convenience and pleasure of refined-flour pasta. They are quick-cooking, easy to prepare, store well, and taste good. Toss one of our sauces on top, and serve with a protein food such as beans, poultry, or fish, add a salad or a green vegetable, and a complete meal is together in a very short time.

Whole-Grain Pasta Cooking Primer

Pasta is a good meal for one, a private little occasion when you can quietly savor a garlicky sauce and the robust flavor of Romano cheese while resting from the day. Pasta meals have many PMS benefits, such as the phytohormones they contain, which modulate your body's estrogen level. Oats, barley, rye, brown rice, whole wheat, and cornmeal all contain these plant hormones.

Whole-grain pastas are usually cooked until tender, not al dente. They need to be cooked a little more so they are easier to digest. Here is a simple technique for cooking whole-grain pasta; any favorite recipe can be converted to this technique.

In a large soup pot, bring 2 quarts purified water to a boil, covered. Add 1 teaspoon sea salt, if using (see Note), and add 8 ounces whole-grain pasta or noodles. Stir and return to a boil, uncovered. Lower flame and cook uncovered until tender (for recommended cooking time read package or taste a strand), 7 to 12 minutes.

Place a large serving bowl in the sink, put a colander in it, and pour the pasta and water into the colander. Lift the colander and shake to drain the excess water. (Do not rinse with water.) Place the colander in the pot to drain further. Allow the hot water to stay in the bowl for 30 to 60 seconds, then discard (or save to use as a soup base). Pour the pasta into the serving bowl, cover with a sauce, and serve immediately.

Note: Salt the water when the pasta does not contain salt, as in Italian and American pastas. Udon and soba, the Japanese pastas, contain salt, and should be cooked without added salt.

Penne Primavera with Tricolored Peppers

Yield: 4 servings   100% vegetarian

We've tossed a rainbow of peppers with garlic to create a dish full of flavor that's easy and fast to prepare.

PMS Benefits: Whole-grain pastas contain the bran, germ, and endosperm and are complex carbohydrates. These whole foods are innately satisfying and tend not to lead to PMS nibbling to maintain steady blood sugar.

2   **quarts purified water**
1   **teaspoon sea salt**
8   **ounces whole wheat penne or fusilli**
4   **tablespoons extra-virgin olive oil**
1   **onion, sliced**
2   **cloves garlic, minced**
1   **red bell pepper, seeded and sliced thin**
1   **green bell pepper, seeded and sliced thin**
· 1   **yellow bell pepper, seeded and sliced thin**
½   **cup homemade salt-free vegetable stock or additional purified water**
¼   **cup pignolia (see Note)**
½   **teaspoon herbal sea salt**
    Pinch ground pepper
4   **sprigs fresh parsley, washed, thick stems removed, and minced**
    Grated Parmesan cheese (optional)

1. In a large soup pot, on high heat, bring the water to a boil, covered. Add the sea salt, penne or fusilli, and stir. Return the water to a boil, uncovered. Lower heat and simmer until tender, 7 to 10 minutes.

2. In a large sauté pan, heat 2 tablespoons olive oil, and stir in the onion and garlic. Cook, covered, on medium heat, until the onion begins to turn translucent, about 5 minutes.

3. Add the red, green, and yellow peppers, and stock or water. Cover and bring the liquid to a boil. Lower heat and cook until the peppers are tender, 5 to 7 minutes. Stir occasionally.

4. Place a serving bowl in the sink and put a colander in it. Carefully pour the cooked pasta into the colander (the hot water will warm the serving bowl). Remove the colander and set it in the pot, to drain further.

5. In a small skillet, toast the pignolia until golden and fragrant. Stir constantly to prevent burning. Once toasted, remove to a nonplastic plate or bowl to cool.

6. Discard the cooking water (or save to use as a soup base) from the serving bowl. Pour the drained pasta into the hot bowl. Add the remaining 2 tablespoons olive oil with the herbal sea salt and pepper.

7. Toss the cooked peppers and parsley in with the pasta. Top with the roasted pignolia and serve with the cheese on the side, if desired. Add a salad for a very satisfying meal.

Cooking Tip: You can roast the peppers instead of sautéing them. Peel the roasted peppers, slice, and add them at the end of the recipe. (See page 59 for instructions on how to roast peppers.)

Note: Pignolia are nuts that come from several varieties of pine trees; the nut is found inside the pinecone. Pignolia-bearing pine trees are found in such diverse regions as China, Italy, and the American southwest. Keep pignolia refrigerated or frozen to preserve the nut oils.

Nutritional Stars: B-complex vitamins, vitamin E, calcium, iron, magnesium, manganese, selenium, zinc

 ## Adolpho's Pasta Fagioli

Yield: 4 to 6 servings   100% vegetarian

This hearty Italian pasta and bean stew was handed down through Lissa's family, and her father taught us how to prepare it. Traditionally, pasta fagioli was made after preparing fresh pasta, to use up the little bits and broken pieces. Serve it thick or soupy, with the addition of a little flaked red pepper and grated pecorino Romano cheese to round off the flavors. It's sure to be a favorite!

PMS Benefits: Beans and whole grains contain quality fiber and are low in fat. Eating these kinds of foods can decrease a woman's estrogen level, which when high, may lead to cramping, excess bleeding, and fibroids. When a diet lower in animal fat is consumed, less estrogen accumulates.

Before you begin, soak ½ cup sorted and washed dried cannellini or Great Northern beans in a bowl with 3 cups purified water for 6 hours or overnight.

(Adolpho's Pasta Fagioli—Continued)

    1 cup soaked cannellini or Great Northern beans (from ½ cup dried beans)
    8 cups purified water plus additional as needed
    1 bay leaf
    ¼ cup extra-virgin olive oil
    4 cloves garlic, minced
    2 stalks celery, ends trimmed, minced
    1 onion, minced
    ½ bunch Italian parsley, washed, thick stems removed, and minced
    1 teaspoon dried basil
    ½ teaspoon dried oregano
    1 or 2 pinches red pepper flakes plus additional as needed
    1 to 2 teaspoons sea salt
    3 ripe plum tomatoes, cores removed, chopped
    ¼ to ½ cup whole-grain pasta, such as broken spaghetti or udon, elbows, ribbons, or shells
    Grated pecorino (sheep's milk) Romano cheese (optional)

1. With your hands or a slotted spoon, remove the beans from the soaking water to a large saucepan. Add the fresh water and bay leaf, cover, and bring to a boil. Lower flame and simmer for 40 minutes. They will be slightly al dente or undercooked.

2. In a large soup pot, on a medium flame, heat 2 tablespoons oil and add the minced garlic, celery, and onion—the *battuto* (see Note). Stir well. Cook on a low flame for 5 minutes.

3. Add the parsley, basil, oregano, pepper flakes, and 1 teaspoon sea salt. Stir well. Cover and cook on a low flame for 5 minutes.

4. Add the tomatoes and stir. Cover and continue cooking on a low flame for 10 to 15 minutes.

5. Add the al dente beans and cooking liquid to the vegetables and cook until the beans are tender, about 15 minutes.

6. In a large saucepan, bring 1 quart water to a boil, covered. Add 1 teaspoon salt, and stir in the pasta. Return to a boil and simmer uncovered, until the pasta is tender, about 10 minutes.

7. Place a colander in the sink and carefully pour in the cooked pasta. Shake the colander to further drain the water from the pasta.

8. Add the cooked pasta to the beans, stir, and cook for another 5 to 7 minutes.

9. Ladle pasta fagioli into wide bowls and garnish with grated cheese, if desired. Place a small dish of red pepper flakes on the table for an additional spicy taste.

Cooking Tip: A *battuto* is a finely minced seasoning mixture made up of onion, garlic, and celery. It can be used in many recipes.

Nutritional Stars: B-complex vitamins, vitamin E, calcium, iron, magnesium, manganese, selenium, zinc

 ## Soba Noodles in Creamy Mushroom Sauce with Golden Garlic Bits

Yield: 4 servings   100% vegetarian

One of our favorite combinations—buckwheat noodles with a rich and creamy sauce. Have some curled up in a big, soft chair with a romantic book to escape the pressures of the day!

PMS Benefits: Flavonoids mimic estrogen and modulate its fluctuations. Their presence in the body helps to ease the psychological symptoms of anxiety, irritability, and mood swings. Buckwheat is the only grain that contains flavonoids.

2 **quarts purified water**
1 **package soba noodles**
1 **recipe Creamy Mushroom Sauce with Golden Garlic Bits**
   (see page 201)
4 **sprigs fresh parsley, washed, thick stems removed, and minced**

1. In a large soup pot, heat the water to a boil, covered. Add the soba (you may want to break them in half) and stir. Return the water to a boil and simmer until tender, 6 to 8 minutes.

2. Place a serving bowl in the sink and put a colander in it. Carefully pour the cooked soba into the colander (this will warm the serving bowl). Lift the colander to drain further. Discard the cooking water (or save to use as a soup base) and pour the drained soba into the serving bowl.

3. Pour the sauce over the soba and toss. Place the parsley on top of the soba. Serve immediately.

Cooking Tip: Soba is available made with 100% buckwheat flour or with some added whole wheat flour, which has a lighter texture and taste. We think that the flavors of soba and tomato sauce don't mix. Instead, enjoy soba with a savory sauce, such as the one in this recipe.

Nutritional Stars: B-complex vitamins, flavonoids, boron, magnesium, manganese

Minted Couscous and Green Pea Timbales

Yield: 4 servings   100% vegetarian

Once cooked, couscous will take the shape of any mold. We've added green peas for color and shaped the mixture in muffin cups.

PMS Benefits: Craving carbohydrates and sweets is your body's attempt to self-medicate PMS anxiety. When carbohydrates are consumed, the body produces more serotonin, which in moderate amounts generates a feeling of calmness and well-being. Complex carbohydrates such as whole grains will provide this feeling without wrecking havoc with your blood sugar.

- 2 cups purified water
- 1 mint-tea bag, or 3 or 4 sprigs fresh mint, leaves only
- 1 cup whole wheat couscous
- 1 teaspoon herbal sea salt
- ½ cup fresh peas or sugar snaps, cut into pea-sized pieces
- 3 tablespoons unsalted butter, preferably organic
- 8 to 12 fresh mint leaves, washed

1. In a medium-sized saucepan, bring the water to a boil, covered. Add the tea bag, couscous, and herbal sea salt (if using fresh mint, chop fine before adding and stir into couscous). Lower flame and simmer for 5 minutes.

2. Using tongs, remove and discard the tea bag. Add the peas or sugar snaps and butter on top of the couscous without stirring. Cover and continue to cook, 5 to 7 minutes.

3. Using a pastry brush, lightly oil the cups of a muffin pan.

4. Using a fork, scratch the surface of the couscous to fluff and separate while stirring in the peas. Spoon the couscous into 8 to 12 muffin cups. Wet your fingers lightly with water or use the back of a spoon, and press the couscous mixture firmly into the muffin cups to shape timbales. When all are formed, place a platter or cutting board over the muffin pan and invert them at the same time. Tap the bottom of the muffin pan with a wooden spoon to loosen.

5. Serve two timbales per person. Place a fresh mint leaf on the top of each. (Or spoon the couscous into a serving bowl and serve hot.)

Nutritional Stars: B-complex vitamins, vitamin E, calcium, iron, magnesium, manganese, selenium, zinc

Nonna Virginia's Fettuccini with Tuna Sauce

Yield: 4 servings

Here's an interesting and fast way to mix the benefits of fish with those of whole grains. Add a few dashes of red pepper flakes to turn up the heat—and mangia!

PMS Benefits: Whole-grain pasta contains a wide variety of nutrients that are good for you all month long. This fettuccini contains vitamins B1, B2, B3, B5, B6, E, folic acid, and inositol. The minerals include calcium, iron, magnesium, and zinc.

2 quarts plus ½ cup purified water
1 teaspoon sea salt
8 ounces whole wheat fettuccini or spaghetti
4 tablespoons extra-virgin olive oil
2 onions, minced
3 cloves garlic, chopped
½ teaspoon herbal sea salt
¼ teaspoon ground pepper
8 ripe tomatoes, cores removed, chopped fine (see Note)
1 to 2 pinches red pepper flakes
2 cans tuna packed in olive oil, preferably imported
4 sprigs fresh parsley, washed, thick stems removed, minced
Grated Parmesan cheese (optional)

1. In a large soup pot, on high heat, bring 2 quarts of water to a boil, covered. Add the salt and fettuccini or spaghetti (you may want to break them in half) and stir. Return the water to a boil, uncovered. Lower heat and simmer until tender, 7 to 10 minutes.

2. In a medium-sized saucepan, heat 2 tablespoons olive oil, and add the onions, garlic, herbal sea salt, and pepper. Sauté on medium heat, uncovered, until the onions begin to turn translucent, about 10 minutes. Stir frequently.

3. Place a serving bowl in the sink and put a colander in it. Carefully pour the cooked pasta into the colander (this will warm the serving bowl). Remove the colander and set in the pot, to drain further.

4. Add the tomatoes, ½ cup water, and red pepper flakes to the saucepan. Stir well. Cover and bring to a boil.

5. Drain the oil from the cans of tuna and add the tuna to the tomato mixture. Return to a boil, covered. Lower heat and cook another 5 minutes.

6. Add the remaining 2 tablespoons olive oil. Taste and add additional salt and pepper, if desired.

7. Discard the cooking water (or save to use as a soup base) from the serving bowl. Pour the drained pasta into the hot bowl. Ladle the tuna sauce on top and toss. Sprinkle the parsley on top. Serve with grated cheese and a small bowl of red pepper flakes, if desired.

Cooking Tip: Whole-grain pasta cooking water is terrific to save and use later as a soup stock or in a stew. It will give the soup or stew a rich flavor. Remember to reduce the amount of salt the recipe calls for, however, since the pasta stock will already be salted.

Note: Instead of the fresh tomatoes and water, one 28-ounce can crushed tomatoes in juice or two boxes Pomi-brand crushed tomatoes may be substituted.

Nutritional Stars: B-complex vitamins, vitamin E, calcium, iron, magnesium, manganese, selenium, zinc

The Doctor Says: "Eat Your Veggies"

One Dozen Leafy Greens

Other Garden Vegetables

Quality Vegetables

When you shop for vegetables, search for fresh rather than frozen or canned. You are more likely to benefit from just-harvested farmer's market produce, since many nutrients begin to degrade once a vegetable or fruit is picked. If your schedule requires that you buy vegetables and cook them several days later, then shop for the longer-lasting root vegetables and tubers such as carrots, parsnips, and potatoes, as well as cabbages and winter squash. Broccoli, asparagus, peppers, and salad greens are far more perishable.

Make a special point of buying produce that is organically grown rather than commercially farmed. We've read enough about the prevalence of toxic chemicals in the food chain and how these can potentially affect our long-term health that eating organic produce is our personal priority. Chemical fertilizers, pesticides, herbicides, and chemical sprays—both those used in the fields and to preserve produce for lengthy storage—stress the liver. Once we take these substances into the body, we must detoxify them. If the liver is overburdened with toxic chemicals, it is less efficient at deactivating hormones, which leads to estrogen/progesterone imbalance, triggering menstrual symptoms. In addition, because organic produce is not treated with preservatives to extend its shelf life, it tends to be fresh-picked and higher in nutrients—a PMS bonus.

How to Wash, Cook, Season, and Store Vegetables

1. How to wash vegetables: We use a natural-fiber vegetable brush (also known as a *tawashi*) and purified water to clean our vegetables. When vegetables are waxed, peeling removes this. Some vegetables have fungicides sprayed on them to give a longer shelf life. Clean these with a mild soap first, then peel them. When using organic vegetables, you don't need to worry about waxes, fungicides, or preservatives.

2. How to cook vegetables: Vegetables that are cut into similar sizes cook evenly. We use many cooking techniques in our vegetable recipes, such as steaming, sautéing, stir-frying, and boiling. A fast way to steam is to put ¼ to ½ inch of water (about ½ to 1 cup) in a saucepan with a tight-fitting lid. Bring the water to a boil and then add the vegetables; steam as usual. A steamer basket can also be used.

   If liquid remains after cooking, drink it as a light bouillon or use it as a stock for another dish such as soup, beans, or grain. Refrigerated, this liquid stores for 3 to 5 days.

3. How to season: Salt after the vegetables are cooked, otherwise the salt can toughen the vegetables and draw out their nutrients.

4. How to store vegetables: Most vegetables do best when stored in plastic bags and placed in the vegetable bin. Mushrooms and ginger do better in paper. Garlic and onions will stay fresh if left on the counter top, away from heat and direct sunlight.

Vegetable Cooking Times

When using a combination of vegetables that cook at different times, cook them separately or layer them in the saucepan, with the vegetable that cooks the longest on the bottom and the one that cooks the least on the top.

Vegetable	Steaming[1]	Blanching/boiling[1]	Baking[1]
Asparagus	10 minutes	8 minutes	15 minutes
Beets	1½ hours	45 minutes	50 minutes
Black radish, diced	20 minutes	15 minutes	20 minutes
Broccoli florets	8 minutes	5 minutes	15 minutes
Bronzini florets	8 minutes	5 minutes	15 minutes
Brussels sprouts	10 minutes	8 minutes	15 minutes
Cabbage, cut into chunks	12 minutes	10 minutes	20 minutes
Carrots, diced	12 minutes	10 minutes	20 minutes
Cauliflower florets	8 minutes	5 minutes	15 minutes
Corn kernels	4 minutes	2 minutes	10 minutes
Daikon, diced	10 minutes	8 minutes	15 minutes
Fennel, diced	10 minutes	8 minutes	15 minutes
Green beans	10 minutes	8 minutes	20 minutes
Kohlrabi, diced	15 minutes	10 minutes	25 minutes
Leeks, chopped	4 minutes	2 minutes	10 minutes
Mushrooms (button)	8 minutes	5 minutes	15 minutes
Onions, diced	10 minutes	8 minutes	20 minutes
Peppers, bell, red and green	10 minutes	8 minutes	15 minutes
Potatoes, diced	12 minutes	10 minutes	25 minutes
Potatoes, whole	—	25 minutes	30 minutes
Snow peas	2 minutes	1 minute	4 minutes
Sugar snaps	2 minutes	1 minute	4 minutes
Sweet potato, diced	12 minutes	10 minutes	25 minutes
Turnips, diced	15 minutes	12 minutes	20 minutes
Yam, diced	12 minutes	10 minutes	25 minutes

[1] These are approximate cooking times, which depend on the size of the vegetable or pieces.

Dark, Leafy Greens: Washing and Cooking Primer

Here are all of the basics you need to know to cook any of the more bitter dark, leafy greens—including broccoli rabe, kale, dandelion and mustard greens, and collards. This does not include spinach, Swiss chard, or beet greens.

1. To wash: Fill a large bowl with cool water. Cut ¼ to ½ inch off the bottom of the stems. (Do not remove the entire stem, unless a recipe specifically calls for it.) Dunk the greens in the water. Remove a few leaves at a time and place in a colander to drain.
2. To cook: In a large soup pot, bring 2 to 3 quarts purified water to a boil, covered. Add the washed greens and, using a wooden spoon, stir them down into the water. Return the pot to a boil, uncovered. Lower flame and simmer until the stems are flexible and easy to pierce with the point of a paring knife, 7 to 10 minutes.
3. To drain: Place a colander in the sink and pour in the cooked greens, discarding the water. Drain well and cool.
4. To chop: Once the greens have cooled, gather the cooked greens in your hands and squeeze them to remove any excess water. At this point chop, season, marinate, bake, roll, etc.

Spinach, Chard, and Beet Greens: Washing and Cooking Primer

These greens require a different method of washing and cooking. Since they tend to be very sandy, they need to be washed more thoroughly. Usually two or three washings are needed to be sure the sand has been removed. Spinach chard and beet greens are also very delicate and require more gentle steaming rather than boiling to soften them.

1. To wash: Trim ½ inch off the stem ends. Fill a large bowl with water. Separate the leaves, push them into the water, dunk them up and down, and swish them around. Remove the leaves from the water and put into a colander. Discard the washing water, rinse the bowl, and repeat at least one more time, until there is no sand left in the bottom of the bowl. The greens are now ready either to cook or to use raw.
2. To cook: Put the washed, wet greens into a large pot. Place on the stove on medium heat and bring to a boil, covered. Lower heat and cook until the greens have wilted. If you are using a thin-bottomed pot, or burners that are hard to regulate, add 1 cup water to the pot before you begin cooking.

3. To drain: Place a colander in the sink. Pour the cooked greens and liquid into the colander, discarding the liquid. Allow the cooked greens to cool.

4. To chop: Once cool, gather the greens in your hands and squeeze any excess liquid from them. Place on a cutting board and chop to desired consistency. They are now ready for seasoning.

 # Kale and Yukon Gold Potatoes with Caramelized Onions

Yield: 4 servings　　　100% vegetarian

Potatoes are a great way to disguise the goodness of greens—a tasty introduction to those who think they don't like them. Of course any potatoes will do, but the Yukon golds add a special sweetness, and many people happily eat them without butter, since their taste is so naturally rich.

PMS Benefits: There are many foods that provide calcium besides dairy—whole grains, beans, fresh vegetables, fruits, nuts, seeds, and fish all have some. Leafy greens such as collards, bok choy, chicory, and dandelion and mustard greens also contain appreciable amounts—90 grams of calcium in a cup of kale. Calcium promotes restful sleep to banish end-of-the-month fatigue.

2　**quarts purified water plus additional if needed**
1　**bunch kale, ends trimmed, washed (see Note)**
2　**tablespoons unsalted butter, preferably organic, or extra-virgin olive oil**
2　**onions, peeled and sliced**
　　Herbal sea salt
　　Ground pepper
3　**Yukon gold potatoes, peeled and cut into large chunks**
4　**cloves garlic, minced**

1. In a large soup pot, bring 2 quarts water to a boil, covered. Add the kale and, using a wooden spoon, stir into the water. Return the pot to a boil, uncovered. Lower flame and simmer until the stems are flexible and easy to pierce with a fork, 7 to 10 minutes. Place a colander in the sink and pour in the cooked kale, discarding the water. Drain well and cool.

2. In a large sauté pan, heat the butter or olive oil and add the onions. Cook uncovered on a medium-high flame until the onion browns, about 10 minutes. Stir frequently. Add a pinch of herbal sea salt and pepper. Remove the onions to a small bowl and set aside.

3. Add 1 cup water to the sauté pan and the potatoes and garlic. Bring to a boil, covered. Reduce the flame and cook until the potatoes are soft when a fork is inserted, 10 to 15 minutes. Season with ½ teaspoon herbal sea salt and ¼ teaspoon pepper. Stir well.

4. In a blender or food processor, pulse-mince the kale or chop fine by hand.

5. Add the kale to the cooked potatoes and stir. And a little water to remove any potato that has stuck to the bottom. Stir gently, being careful not to break up the potatoes too much.

6. Spoon the vegetables into a serving bowl. Top with the caramelized onions and serve hot.

Cooking Tip: We like using a timer that clips to your apron or fits in a pocket. When you walk out of the kitchen you'll be less likely to forget there is something cooking—no more scorched saucepans or overcooked vegetables.

Note: Collard, dandelion, or mustard greens can be used instead of kale.

Nutritional Stars: Vitamin B6, beta-carotene, folic acid, vitamin E, calcium, iron, magnesium, omega-3 fatty acids

Italian Broccoli Rabe with Stewed Tomatoes and Black Olives

Yield: 4 servings   100% vegetarian

This dish is great in the late summer and early fall when tomatoes are at their peak and the broccoli rabe is newly harvested and young. Look for bunches with tightly closed flowers.

PMS Benefits: It's easy to spot foods that contain beta-carotene, a natural orange pigment in vegetables such as butternut squash and tomatoes. However, this important vitamin, a precursor to vitamin A, is also in green vegetables such as spinach, kale, and broccoli rabe, but masked by the green of chlorophyll. Vitamin A helps prevent fluid retention and premenstrual weight gain.

(Italian Broccoli Rabe with Stewed Tomatoes and Black Olives—Continued)

  3 **tablespoons extra-virgin olive oil**
  1 **onion, chopped**
 10 **cloves garlic, sliced**
  3 **ripe beefsteak or 6 plum tomatoes, cores removed, chopped**
  5 **unsulphured raisins**
 ½ **cup purified water**
 ½ **teaspoon sea salt**
 ¼ **teaspoon ground pepper**
  1 **bunch broccoli rabe, bottoms trimmed, washed**
    Pinch red pepper flakes or cayenne pepper
  8 **to 10 oil-cured black olives, pits removed, chopped**

1. In a large skillet, heat the oil and add the onion. Cook on medium heat, covered, until the onion becomes translucent, 5 to 7 minutes. Stir occasionally.

2. Add the garlic, tomatoes, raisins, water, salt, and pepper. Cook, covered, on a medium-low flame until the tomatoes start to fall apart, 15 to 20 minutes.

3. Chop the broccoli rabe coarsely and add to the cooking tomatoes with the red pepper flakes. Stir well. Cover and cook on medium heat until the greens wilt, 5 to 7 minutes.

4. Add the olives, stir, and cook another 1 or 2 minutes. Add a little water if the tomatoes are drying and sticking to the bottom. (It should be saucelike.)

5. Spoon the cooked broccoli rabe and tomatoes into a large ceramic platter or bowl and serve with a small bowl of red pepper flakes on the side.

Cooking Tip: Sun-dried tomatoes can be used instead of fresh ones—substitute fresh tomatoes in this recipe with ¾ cup reconstituted sun-dried tomatoes and an additional ½ cup purified water.

Nutritional Stars: Vitamin A, vitamin B6, folic acid, vitamin E, calcium, iron, magnesium, omega-3 fatty acids

Spinach and Sweet Potato Sauté

Yield: 4 servings   100% vegetarian

Dark spinach and shimmering sweet potatoes make a great color combination and flavor duo—bitter meets sweet.

PMS Benefits: Spinach is like a multivitamin and mineral supplement in a green leaf. It contains therapeutic levels of vitamin A, vitamin B6, folic acid, iron, and magnesium, as well as many other PMS-friendly nutrients.

1½ **cups purified water**
2 **sweet potatoes or yams, peeled and cut into chunks**
1 **bunch spinach, ends trimmed, washed (see page 107)**
2 **tablespoons unsalted butter, preferably organic, or extra-virgin olive oil**
½ **teaspoon herbal sea salt**
¼ **teaspoon ground white pepper**
2 **cloves garlic, minced**

1. In a medium-sized sauté pan, bring 1 cup water to a boil. Add the sweet potatoes or yams and cover. Cook until soft when pierced with a fork, about 10 minutes.

2. In a medium-sized saucepan, bring ½ cup water to a boil. Add the spinach and cook until it wilts, 4 to 5 minutes. Place a colander in the sink and pour in the cooked spinach. Drain and allow to cool.

3. Gather the spinach in your hands and squeeze to remove excess water. Chop and add to the yams. Add the butter or oil, herbal sea salt, and pepper. Stir well, and cook uncovered until all of the water evaporates, 3 to 4 minutes. Add the garlic and cook another 1 or 2 minutes.

4. Taste and sprinkle additional seasoning, if desired.

Cooking Tip: To produce unsalted butter, the manufacturer uses fresher cream to insure that the delicate taste is sweet.

Nutritional Stars: Vitamin A, vitamin B6, vitamin E, magnesium

Red Chard Patties

Yield: 4 servings   100% vegetarian

You can find green or red Swiss chard. Greengrocers also refer to this leafy vege-
table simply as "chard," another name for this delicious and mineral-rich green.

PMS Benefits: Swiss chard is rich in folic acid, one of the B vitamins that are
essential to the PMS menu. It aids in the production of red blood cells, preventing
anemia. As heavy menstrual flow can lead to anemia and fatigue, it is especially important to maintain healthy levels of this B vitamin.

- 2 **bunches red or green chard, ends trimmed, washed (see Note)**
- 1 **cup purified water**
- 1 **egg, preferably organic**
- 1 **onion, minced or grated**
- 2 **cloves garlic, minced**
- ¼ **to ½ cup whole-grain bread crumbs**
- 1 **teaspoon herbal sea salt**
- ¼ **teaspoon ground white pepper**
- ⅛ **teaspoon nutmeg**
- 4 **tablespoons unsalted butter, preferably organic, or ghee (see page 227)**
- 4 **tablespoons extra-virgin olive oil**
- 1 **lemon, cut into wedges**

1. Put the chard and water into a large soup pot, cover, and bring to a boil.
Reduce flame and cook until the chard wilts, 5 to 7 minutes. Place a colander in
the sink and pour in the chard, discarding the cooking liquid. Allow it to drain well
and cool.

2. Gather the chard into two or three handfuls and squeeze each to remove any
excess water. Chop fine by hand or use a food processor. Place in a medium-sized
bowl and add the egg, onion, garlic, ¼ cup bread crumbs, herbal sea salt, pepper, and
nutmeg. Mix well. Add additional bread crumbs if the mixture is runny or loose.

3. Heat a large skillet with 2 tablespoons butter or ghee and 2 tablespoons olive
oil. The fat should cover the bottom in a thin layer. Using two tablespoons, scoop up
some of the chard mixture in one, and press it down with the other to make a small
oval patty. Slide it off the spoon by pushing it with the second spoon into the hot fat.
Repeat until the skillet is full. Do not overcrowd.

4. Cook until the patty has solidified and holds together, and is golden on the
cooking side. Using two forks, slide one underneath the patty and lift it up to flip

over. Use the second fork to steady the patty and prevent the fat from spattering. Continue to cook until the other side is golden.

5. Using the forks, remove the patties to a brown bag or paper toweling to drain. Place in a warm oven. Repeat with the remaining mixture, butter or ghee, and olive oil, until all of the patties have been cooked.

6. Serve with wedges of lemon.

Cooking Tip: These patties are lightly sautéed in butter, ghee, or olive oil. We prefer a combination of butter or ghee with olive oil in equal proportions.

Note: Spinach or beet greens can be substituted for the chard.

Nutritional Stars: Folic acid, calcium, omega-3 fatty acids

 ## Turnip Greens Chiffonade, Mashed Potatoes, and Ginger

Yield: 4 servings   100% vegetarian

A chiffonade cut (see Cooking Tip 1, page 40) gives these greens a delicate and lacy look—a more luxurious appearance than the original leaves.

PMS Benefits: Rich in calcium, folic acid, and beta-carotene, turnip greens also have fiber, which helps to excrete excess estrogen. Elevated estrogen levels can bring on PMS anxiety, irritability, and mood swings.

    Purified water
  1 bunch turnip greens, ends trimmed, washed
  3 large potatoes, peeled and cut into chunks
  3 tablespoons unsalted butter, preferably organic
  1 1-inch piece fresh ginger, grated
  1 teaspoon herbal sea salt plus additional as needed
  ¼ teaspoon ground white pepper
  2 tablespoons flaxseed oil or extra-virgin olive oil
  1 tablespoon cider or brown rice vinegar

1. In a large soup pot, bring 2 quarts water to a boil, covered. Add the greens and return to a boil, uncovered. Cook until the greens begin to soften, 7 to 10 minutes. Place a colander in the sink, and drain the greens, discarding the liquid. Set aside to cool.

(Turnip Greens Chiffonade, Mashed Potatoes, and Ginger—Continued)

2. Put the potatoes in a large saucepan with enough water to almost cover. Bring to a boil, covered, reduce flame, and cook until soft when pierced with a fork, about 15 minutes.

3. With a slotted spoon, remove the cooked potatoes to a large bowl. Using a potato masher, mash the hot potatoes (or puree in a food processor) until all the lumps are gone. Add the cooking liquid in ½-cup amounts, using as much as needed to soften the potatoes and give a velvety texture.

4. Add the butter and stir to melt. (The potatoes can be returned to the saucepan to be reheated if they are preferred very hot.)

5. Gather the grated ginger in your fingers and over a cup or plate, squeeze the ginger juice from the pulp. Discard the pulp. Add the juice to the potatoes, with the herbal sea salt and pepper. Cover the pot and keep warm.

6. Cut the cooked greens in lacy, thin chiffonade strips (see Cooking Tip 1, page 40). Place in a bowl and sprinkle with a few pinches of herbal sea salt, oil, and vinegar. Stir well. Fold into the potatoes just before serving.

Nutritional Stars: Vitamin A, B-complex vitamins, folic acid, calcium

 ## Mustard Greens au Gratin with Roasted Pignolia

Yield: 4 servings   100% vegetarian

Cream sauces are always a hit with our families. Here we've added chopped greens and topped the dish with pine nuts, which taste divine when roasted.

PMS Benefits: Certain plants contain compounds called phytohormones that function like hormones and help balance those made by the body. This cuts down on PMS symptoms associated with excess estrogen, such as anxiety. The mustard greens in this recipe are a good source of phytohormones.

> 2 **quarts purified water**
> 1 **bunch mustard greens, ends trimmed,washed (see Note)**
> ¼ **cup unsalted butter, preferably organic, ghee (see page 227), or**
>   **extra-virgin olive oil**
> ¼ **cup whole-grain flour**

2 to 3 cups homemade salt-free vegetable stock or additional
   purified water
½ teaspoon herbal sea salt plus additional as needed
¼ teaspoon ground white pepper
10 Greek olives, pitted and sliced, or 2 tablespoons drained capers
½ cup pignolia
½ cup whole-grain bread crumbs
   Grated zest of 1 orange, preferably organic

1. In a large soup pot, bring the water to a boil, covered. Add the greens, and with a wooden spoon, stir them into the water. Return the pot to a boil, uncovered, and cook until the greens begin to soften, 7 to 10 minutes. Place a colander in the sink and drain the greens, discarding the water. Set aside to cool.

2. Meanwhile, in a medium-sized skillet on a moderate flame, heat the butter, ghee, or olive oil with the flour until the mixture is toasty smelling and slightly golden, 4 to 5 minutes. Stir constantly to prevent burning.

3. Add the stock or water to the skillet, in ½-cup amounts, while continuing to stir. Continue to add the liquid until a thick sauce has formed. Add the herbal sea salt and pepper, and cook another minute.

4. Position the oven shelves for an 8 × 8-inch-deep baking dish. Preheat the oven to 350 degrees. Grease an oven-to-table dish with a thin coating of olive oil or butter.

5. Gather the mustard greens into two or three handfuls and squeeze them to remove any excess water. Place on a cutting board and chop coarsely or use a food processor and pulse-chop. Add the greens to the sauce with the olives or capers, and stir well.

6. Pour the mixture into the greased baking dish. In a small bowl, combine the pignolia, bread crumbs, orange zest, several pinches of herbal sea salt, and white pepper. Top the greens mixture with the pignolia combination. Place in the oven and bake until the nuts are toasted and golden, about 20 minutes.

7. Place a trivet on the table for the baking dish. Add a serving spoon and dig in!

Cooking Tip: In this recipe you will learn how to prepare a roux and then a creamy sauce, which are the main components of an au gratin sauce. Using butter or ghee will produce a richer flavor.

Note: Any other dark, leafy greens, such as kale or collards, can be substituted for the mustard greens.

Nutritional Stars: Vitamin C, folic acid, calcium, omega-3 fatty acids

Pickled Collards with Capers, Currants, and Walnuts

Yield: 4 to 6 servings   100% vegetarian

Sweet and sour, salty and spicy—this dish aims to please your palate and curb your PMS cravings. Try it stuffed into a whole-grain pita-pocket bread—we find it irresistible!

PMS Benefits: Collards and other dark, leafy greens are a rich source of omega-3 fatty acids, which are the raw material from which your body produces prostaglandins—hormonelike compounds that ease menstrual cramps.

- 2 **quarts purified water**
- 1 **bunch collard greens, ends trimmed, washed**
- ½ **cup raw walnuts or toasted almonds, chopped coarsely**
- 3 **tablespoons extra-virgin olive oil**
- 2 **tablespoons flaxseed oil**
- 2 **tablespoons capers (optional)**
- 2 **tablespoons unsulphured currants**
  Juice of 1 lemon (3 to 4 tablespoons) or 3 tablespoons cider vinegar
- 1 **clove garlic, minced**
- ¼ **to ½ teaspoon herbal sea salt**

1. In a large soup pot, bring the water to a boil, covered. Add the greens and, using a wooden spoon, stir them into the water. Return the pot to a boil, uncovered, lower flame and simmer until the greens begin to soften, about 10 minutes. Place a colander in the sink and drain the greens, discarding the liquid. Set aside to cool.

2. In a large bowl, mix together the walnuts or almonds, olive and flaxseed oils, capers, currants, lemon juice or vinegar, garlic, and herbal sea salt.

3. Gather the collards into two or three handfuls and squeeze them to remove any excess water. Place on a cutting board and either chop coarsely, fine, or chiffonade (see Cooking Tip 1, page 40). Add to the bowl with the walnut mixture, and stir well.

4. Allow the collards to sit at least 10 minutes to absorb the flavorings, before serving.

Cooking Tip: The most popular variety of walnuts are English and black walnuts, available year-round, either shelled or unshelled. Look for shelled nuts that are meaty, plump, and crisp. Since nuts have a high fat content, store shelled nutmeats in the refrigerator for up to 6 months or in the freezer for up to 1 year.

Nutritional Stars: Vitamin A, vitamin E, calcium, omega-3 fatty acids

Dandelion Greens with Sun-dried Tomatoes and Whole Garlic Cloves

Yield: 4 servings   100% vegetarian

Two of our favorite ingredients—sun-dried tomatoes and whole cloves of garlic— complement these greens and tame their bitterness. Even our husbands eat this one!

PMS Benefits: Vitamin A treats PMS-related skin disorders, including acne. It is an antioxidant, helping to protect the cells, enhance immunity, and slow the aging process. A deficiency of vitamin A results in dry hair and skin and, over time, poor vision at night. Leafy green vegetables such as these dandelion greens are good sources of this versatile vitamin.

½ **cup unsulphured sun-dried tomatoes**
1 **cup plus 2 quarts purified water**
1 **bunch dandelion greens, ends trimmed, washed**
3 **tablespoons extra-virgin olive oil**
10 **to 12 cloves garlic, peeled**
½ **teaspoon sea salt**
   Pinch ground pepper
1 **or 2 tablespoons brown-rice or cider vinegar**

1. In a small saucepan, bring the sun-dried tomatoes and 1 cup water to a boil, covered. Reduce flame and simmer 5 minutes. Turn off flame and set aside.

2. In a large soup pot, bring the 2 quarts water to a boil. Add the greens and return to a boil, uncovered. Lower flame and simmer for 5 minutes. Place a colander in the sink and drain the dandelions, discarding the cooking water. Set aside to cool.

3. Using a sieve, drain the sun-dried tomatoes, discarding the cooking water.

4. Heat a large skillet with the olive oil and add the whole cloves of garlic. Cook on medium heat, stirring frequently, until golden brown, 5 to 7 minutes.

5. Add the tomatoes to the garlic. Quickly cover to avoid splattering. Lower heat and cook for 1 minute.

6. Gather the greens in your hands and squeeze the excess water from them. Chop the dandelions and add to the garlic and tomatoes. Stir well, and season with salt and pepper. Sprinkle the vinegar on and cover. Steam another 2 minutes. Serve hot or at room temperature.

(Dandelion Greens with Sun-dried Tomatoes and Whole Garlic Cloves—Continued)
Cooking Tip: Unsulphured sun-dried tomatoes are dried naturally in the sun. Their color is darker than the sulphured ones, which are bright orange-red and which bear little resemblance to the original vegetable. Their added sulphur, which can cause an allergic reaction, is unnecessary.
Nutritional Stars: Vitamin A, calcium, magnesium, omega-3 fatty acids

 # French Leek, Broccoli, and Potato Quiche

Yield: 4 to 6 servings   100% vegetarian

Visualize yourself sitting in a café along the Seine as you munch this quiche. Music, waiters in black and white, a salad of baby greens, a baguette with fresh beurre. . . .

PMS Benefits: Onions supply selenium, a mineral that may be unfamiliar to some. It functions in tandem with vitamin E, known to reduce menstrual irritability, anxiety, and depression.

2   **tablespoons unsalted butter, preferably organic, or extra-virgin olive oil**
2   **white or yellow onions, sliced**
1   **red onion, sliced**
2   **leeks, white and 3 inches only of green parts, split, washed, and**
       sliced (see page 31)
2   **shallots, sliced**
1   **tablespoon fresh or 1 teaspoon dried marjoram or basil**
½   **teaspoon herbal sea salt**
¼   **teaspoon ground pepper**
3   **eggs, preferably organic**
¼   **cup plain yogurt or buttermilk with living cultures,**
       preferably organic
1   **stalk broccoli, ends trimmed and stalk peeled**
1   **prepared whole wheat piecrust, unbaked**
2   **potatoes, peeled and sliced thin**
6   **sprigs fresh parsley, washed, thick stems removed, and minced**
       Grated Parmesan or Romano cheese, preferably organic (optional)

1. In a large skillet, on a medium-high flame, heat the butter or oil. Sauté the onions until they just begin to turn brown, about 10 minutes. Stir often.

2. Add the leeks, shallots, marjoram or basil, herbal sea salt, and pepper to the skillet and stir well. Cook for 2 minutes.

3. Transfer the leek mixture to a large platter or bowl and cool completely. (This will prevent the egg mixture from cooking and making lumps when mixed in.)

4. Position the oven shelves to fit a deep 9-inch pie pan. Preheat the oven to 425 degrees.

5. In a blender or using a whisk in a medium-sized bowl, beat the eggs and yogurt or buttermilk. Chop the broccoli stalk and florets.

6. Place the piecrust on a baking sheet. In the piecrust, arrange half of the potatoes in a layer and top with the broccoli. Pour one-third of the egg mixture over. Spread a single thick layer of the leek mixture on top of the broccoli and pour another one-third of the egg mixture over. Top with the remaining potatoes. Stir the parsley into the remaining egg mixture. Slowly pour it on top of the final potato layer.

7. Carefully place the quiche in the oven. Bake for 10 minutes at 425 degrees. Lower the heat to 350 degrees and bake for another 30 to 35 minutes or until the eggs are set and the crust is golden brown. If using cheese, sprinkle some over the top during the last 10 minutes of baking, allowing it to melt.

8. Allow the quiche to cool about 5 minutes before cutting, to settle and firm up. Cut into wedges and serve while still warm.

Cooking Tip: Prepared whole wheat piecrusts are available in the frozen section at the natural-food store. If they aren't available, make a crustless quiche by buttering the pie pan and sprinkling it with whole-grain bread crumbs. Pour in the filling and bake as usual.

Nutritional Stars: Vitamin A, vitamin B6, vitamin C, flavonoids, magnesium

 # Pureed Brussels Sprouts with Yogurt, Cumin, and Nutmeg

Yield: 4 servings   100% vegetarian

In this recipe, Brussels sprouts are treated to creamy yogurt, the faintly exotic scent of cumin, and earthy nutmeg.

PMS Benefits: Brussels sprouts are a good source of the B-complex vitamins that can help women with PMS withstand daily stress. They also contain fiber, which when added to the friendly bacteria in the yogurt, promotes intestinal health and absorption of these needed nutrients.

(Pureed Brussels Sprouts with Yogurt, Cumin, and Nutmeg—Continued)

 1 **cup purified water**
 2 **pints Brussels sprouts, ends trimmed, washed**
 ¼ **teaspoon sea salt**
 1 **cup plain yogurt with active cultures, preferably organic**
 ½ **to 1 teaspoon cumin powder**
 ¼ **teaspoon nutmeg**
 ¼ **teaspoon herbal sea salt**
 ¼ **teaspoon ground white pepper**
 4 **sprigs fresh cilantro (coriander), washed, thick stems removed,
     and chopped coarsely**

 1. In a medium-sized saucepan, bring the water to a boil, covered. Add the Brussels sprouts and sea salt, and return to a boil. Reduce flame and simmer until soft when pierced with a fork, 10 to 12 minutes.

 2. Place a colander in the sink. Pour in the cooked sprouts and drain well, discarding the water. Set aside to cool.

 3. In a blender or food processor, put the sprouts, yogurt, cumin, nutmeg, herbal sea salt, and pepper. Puree until smooth.

 4. Return the mixture to the saucepan and add the cilantro. Heat on low, covered, until warm, about 5 minutes. Serve immediately.

 Cooking Tip: Pureeing in a blender usually requires the addition of a little more liquid than pureeing in a food processor. If there isn't enough liquid for the recipe, add some water.

 Nutritional Stars: B-complex vitamins, vitamin B12, calcium, omega-3 fatty acids

Ukrainian Cabbage and Potatoes
with Fresh Herbs

Yield: 4 servings   100% vegetarian

Here is a novel way to include cabbage in your meals. As the cabbage cooks and turns golden brown, it becomes quite sweet and adds a terrific complement to potatoes—these two ordinary vegetables become extraordinary!

 PMS Benefits: In the nineteenth century in America, the two most commonly eaten vegetables were cabbage and potatoes. Both contain phytoestrogens in small but measurable amounts. Phytoestrogens augment and balance female hormones.

2 tablespoons extra-virgin olive oil
1 onion, sliced
4 cloves garlic, minced
½ head green cabbage, core removed, shredded
2 teaspoons herbal sea salt
1 teaspoon dried oregano
4 potatoes, peeled and quartered
1 cup homemade salt-free vegetable stock or purified water
½ bunch parsley, washed, thick stems removed, and chopped coarsely

1. In a large sauté pan, heat the olive oil and add the onion. Cook, uncovered, over medium-high heat for 3 or 4 minutes, until the onion begins to become translucent.

2. Add the garlic, cabbage, herbal sea salt, and oregano. Continue cooking, covered. Stir occasionally, cooking until the cabbage wilts, about 5 minutes.

3. Add the potatoes and stock or water to the cabbage mixture. Cover and continue cooking over medium heat until the potatoes have softened, 10 to 12 minutes. Uncover and cook another 5 minutes, until the cabbage starts to brown. Add the parsley and stir well.

Cooking Tip: If peeling onions makes you cry, cold onions will make your eyes tear less! Store some onions in the refrigerator.

Nutritional Stars: Vitamin C, folic acid, vitamin K, magnesium, manganese, omega-3 fatty acids

Bok Choy and Shiitake Mushrooms in Chinese Black Bean Sauce

Yield: 4 servings   100% vegetarian

Stir-frying techniques, as in this recipe, are good to know for days when you need quick-cooking methods. Tossed a few times in a wok or sauté pan, the delicious foods you are cooking will fill your kitchen with tempting aromas.

PMS Benefits: This dish is high in vitamin C, a nutrient quickly depleted by stress. Low stores of vitamin C can bring on premenstrual fatigue.

(Bok Choy and Shiitake Mushrooms in Chinese Black Bean Sauce—Continued)

  6 **to 8 shiitake mushrooms**
1¼ **cup plus 2 tablespoons purified water**
  3 **tablespoons fermented black beans (see page 225)**
  2 **tablespoons unrefined sesame or extra-virgin olive oil**
  1 **onion, sliced**
  3 **cloves garlic, minced**
  1 **medium bunch bok choy**
  1 **cup homemade salt-free vegetable stock or additional purified water**
  1 **to 2 tablespoons soy sauce**
  1 **tablespoon arrowroot or kuzu powder (see page 228)**
  2 **teaspoons dark sesame oil**
  4 **sprigs fresh cilantro (coriander), washed, thick stems removed,**
       and chopped coarsely

1. In a small bowl, soak the mushrooms in 1 cup water for about 10 minutes.

2. In a small saucepan, bring ¼ cup water to boil. Turn off flame and add the fermented black beans. Set aside to soak and cool for 10 to 15 minutes.

3. Heat the 2 tablespoons water and sesame or olive oil in a wok or sauté pan. Add the onion and cook for 1 minute. Add garlic and cook for another 30 seconds.

4. Slice the bok choy stems into ¼-inch pieces, and the green leaves into ½-inch pieces; reserve them in separate bowls. Squeeze the water from the soaking mushrooms. Remove the stems and discard. Slice the mushrooms caps thin. Add to the onion and garlic with ½ cup stock or water. Cook covered for 5 to 7 minutes.

5. Add the bok choy stems to the pan and stir. Cover and cook for 3 minutes.

6. Drain the soaking black beans, discarding the liquid. Place in a small bowl with the soy sauce, arrowroot or kuzu, and remaining ½ cup stock or water. Mash with a fork or the back of a spoon, mixing well.

7. Increase the heat to high. Add the bok choy leaves and black-bean mixture to the pan, stirring well. Cook until the liquid has thickened and is clear. Cook 30 seconds more.

8. Add the dark sesame oil and cilantro, stirring once more.

Cooking Tip: When cooking in a wok or sauté pan, put the water in the pan first, then the oil. This will keep the temperature to 212 degrees and reduce the risk of the oil breaking down at higher temperatures, producing toxic substances.

Nutritional Stars: Vitamin A, vitamin B3, vitamin B6, vitamin C, folic acid

Butternut Squash Whip with Roasted Cinnamon-Almonds

Yield: 4 servings   100% vegetarian

Pureed food eases PMS tensions, and we find this dish one of our favorites for that time of the month.

PMS Benefits: Butternut squash and other deep-orange vegetables are a rich source of beta-carotene, the precursor to vitamin A, which encourages skin growth and prevents menstrual bloating.

- 1 **butternut squash, peeled, seeded, and cut into chunks**
- 4 **cloves garlic, minced**
- 2 **apples, cores removed, quartered**
- 1 **onion, quartered**
- 1 **cup unsweetened apple juice or purified water**
- 3 **tablespoons unsalted butter, preferably organic**
- ½ **teaspoon sea salt plus additional as needed**
- 2 **tablespoons ghee (see page 227) or additional unsalted butter, preferably organic**
- ½ **cup raw almonds**
- ½ **teaspoon cinnamon**
- 2 **tablespoons pure maple syrup (optional)**

1. In a large saucepan, put the butternut squash, garlic, apples, onion, and juice or water. Bring to a boil, covered. Reduce flame and simmer until the squash is tender when pierced with a fork, about 20 minutes.

2. With a slotted spoon, remove the squash mixture from the saucepan to a blender or food processor. Add half of the liquid with the butter and ½ teaspoon salt. Puree until smooth. Add more liquid if needed to keep the machine pureeing. With a rubber spatula, scoop the puree into a ceramic bowl. Cover to keep warm.

3. In a medium-sized skillet, melt the ghee or butter and add the almonds, cinnamon, and a pinch of salt. Cook until slightly golden, about 5 minutes, stirring frequently. Be careful not to burn. Remove to a plate to cool.

4. Chop the almonds coarsely. Place in a small bowl and mix with the maple syrup, if a sweeter taste is desired. Garnish the top of the squash puree with the Roasted Cinnamon-Almonds, and serve as a starter to a wonderful homemade meal.

Cooking Tip: If the apples and butternut squash are not organic, please peel them to remove the wax.

Nutritional Stars: Vitamin A, vitamin B2, calcium

Roasted Garden Vegetables au Papillotte

Yield: 4 to 6 servings   100% vegetarian

Parchment paper is an amazing and easy-to-use cooking tool. Wrap any vegetable, fish, or poultry in parchment paper and you'll have moist and fully baked foods—a delight to the clean-up crew!

PMS Benefits: Fresh vegetables are a great source of fiber, which sweeps estrogen out of your body and lessens such PMS symptoms as anxiety.

> 2 **onions, cut into chunks (see Note)**
> 2 **beets or 2 carrots, ends trimmed, cut into chunks**
> 4 **to 6 cloves garlic, peeled**
> 1 **white turnip, ends trimmed, cut into chunks**
> 1 **parsnip, ends trimmed, cut into chunks**
> ½ **rutabaga, peeled and cut into chunks**
> 2 **tablespoons extra-virgin olive oil**
> 1 **teaspoon dried basil**
> ½ **teaspoon dried sage or marjoram**
> ½ **teaspoon herbal sea salt**
> ¼ **teaspoon ground pepper**
>   **Juice of ½ lemon or a splash cider vinegar (optional)**
>   **Parchment paper**

1. In a large bowl, put the onions, beets or carrots, garlic, turnip, parsnip, and rutabaga, and toss with the olive oil, basil, sage or marjoram, herbal sea salt, and pepper. Add the lemon juice or splash with the vinegar, and stir again.

2. Position the oven shelves to fit a baking sheet in the center. Preheat the oven to 350 degrees.

3. Cut four to six sheets of parchment paper into 1-foot lengths. Place the paper on a work surface and divide the seasoned vegetables evenly among the sheets, making sure a clove of garlic is in each. Close the packages by gathering up the corners and twisting tightly at the top.

4. Place the packages on a baking sheet and bake for 30 minutes.

5. Open one package to test the vegetables—they should be tender when pierced with a fork and moist. Place the packages on a serving platter. Allow each person to take one when ready.

Cooking Tip: Parchment paper eliminates the need to grease baking pans, pie plates, and other baking utensils. It can also be used to cover foods or wrap them, as we do here, and bake directly in the paper, preserving the flavors and juices.

Note: Add other favorite vegetables, such as black radishes, daikon, kohlrabi, potatoes, or yams.

Nutritional Stars: Vitamin A, folic acid, calcium, iron

 # Skillet-roasted Sweet Potatoes, Carrots, and Parsnips with Rosemary

Yield: 4 servings   100% vegetarian

While you preheat the oven, start this recipe on top of the stove in an ovenproof cast-iron or enamel-covered skillet, then transfer the skillet to the oven. The baking will leave the vegetables lightly caramelized and golden brown—and so sweet and tasty—and you can carry the pan directly from the oven to the table.

PMS Benefits: Sweet potatoes and carrots contain carotenoids, which are vitamin A precursors that help prevent menstrual bloating.

2 **tablespoons unsalted butter, preferably organic, or extra-virgin olive oil**
2 **onions, chopped**
1 **bulb garlic, cloves peeled**
2 **parsnips, ends trimmed, chopped**
1 **sweet potato or yam, peeled and cut into chunks**
1 **carrot, ends trimmed, chopped**
2 **teaspoons dried or 3 sprigs fresh rosemary**
½ **teaspoon herbal sea salt**
1 **cup purified water or homemade salt-free vegetable stock**

1. Position the oven shelves to fit the skillet. Preheat the oven to 350 degrees.

2. In a medium-sized or large ovenproof skillet on the stove top, heat the butter or olive oil. Add the onions and garlic cloves. Sauté on medium-high heat, until the onions begin to turn brown on the edges, 5 to 7 minutes.

3. Add the parsnips, sweet potato or yam, carrot, rosemary, and herbal sea salt. Stir well. Cook for 5 minutes on a medium flame.

4. Add the water or stock and stir. Place the skillet in the oven, uncovered. Bake until the vegetables begin to turn golden and the liquid is almost dry, 20 to 30 minutes. Stir once halfway through baking.

(Skillet-roasted Sweet Potatoes, Carrots, and Parsnips with Rosemary—Continued)

5. Place a large trivet on the table for the skillet. Add a serving spoon and serve directly from the skillet.

Cooking Tip: Choose small or medium parsnips for a sweeter taste and less fibrous interior.

Nutritional Stars: Vitamin A, folic acid, calcium

 # Mushroom Cakes

Yield: 4 servings   100% vegetarian

Our version of potato latkes—full of mushrooms with all of their woodsy greatness.

PMS Benefits: Mushrooms of all kinds are the only vegetable that contains appreciable amounts of pantothenic acid (vitamin B5). This antistress vitamin has an important role in the production of the adrenal hormones that help to maintain proper fluid balance—and eliminate PMS bloating!

  2 **eggs, preferably organic**
  3 **potatoes, peeled and grated**
10 **mushrooms, minced**
  2 **cloves garlic, minced**
  1 **onion, grated**
  4 **sprigs fresh parsley, washed, thick stems removed, and minced**
  ½ **teaspoon sea salt**
  ¼ **teaspoon ground pepper**
  ¼ **to ½ cup whole-grain bread crumbs**
  ½ **cup ghee (see page 227) or unsalted butter, preferably organic**
  ½ **cup extra-virgin olive oil**
  ½ **lemon, cut into wedges, or several splashes cider vinegar**

1. In a medium-sized bowl, beat the eggs. Add the potatoes, mushrooms, garlic, onion, parsley, salt, and pepper. Stir well.

2. Add ¼ cup bread crumbs and stir. Set mixture aside for several minutes to absorb the liquid.

3. Meanwhile, heat ¼ cup ghee or butter and ¼ cup olive oil in a large skillet.

4. Stir the potato mixture and if it's still loose or runny, add additional bread crumbs. Stir again.

5. Using two tablespoons, fill one with the potato mixture and use the other to push the mixture into the hot pan. The patty should be 2 to 3 inches in diameter.

6. Cook on medium heat until golden brown. Using two forks, slide one under the patty and flip it over, using the second to steady and help turn it. (This method keeps the patties from splashing hot fat.) Continue cooking until the other side is golden brown.

7. Remove the cooked patties to a brown bag or paper toweling. Add more ghee and olive oil as needed. Continue until all of the potato mixture has been used. Serve with a lemon wedge or a splash of vinegar.

Cooking Tip: Grate the mushrooms and potatoes in the food processor.
Nutritional Stars: Vitamin B2, vitamin B3, vitamin B5, zinc

 # Baked Asparagus Spears with Garlic

Yield: 4 servings   100% vegetarian

Baking asparagus will yield these incredible spears . . . watch them disappear.

PMS Benefits: Vitamin E is known to relieve breast tenderness. Vitamin E is found in whole grains, nuts and seeds, many fish, and some vegetables such as sweet potatoes, asparagus, and cucumbers.

 3 **tablespoons extra-virgin olive oil**
 1 **pound asparagus (see Note)**
 ¼ **cup purified water**
 ½ **cup whole-grain bread crumbs**
 ¼ **cup raw sunflower seeds**
 ½ **teaspoon dried oregano or basil**
 3 **cloves garlic, minced**
 ½ **teaspoon herbal sea salt**
 ¼ **teaspoon ground white pepper**

1. Position the oven rack to fit a baking pan. Preheat the oven to 350 degrees.

2. Oil the bottom of the baking pan with 2 teaspoons of the oil. Break the thick stems off the asparagus and discard. Put the asparagus into the baking pan with the water.

3. In a small bowl, mix the bread crumbs, sunflower seeds, oregano or basil, garlic, herbal salt, and pepper with the remaining oil. Sprinkle the crumb mixture

(Baked Asparagus Spears with Garlic—Continued)
over the asparagus. Put the pan in the oven and bake 20 minutes, uncovered. The crumbs will be golden brown.

4. Put a trivet on the table and serve directly from the pan or, using a large spatula, carefully remove the asparagus to a platter and serve hot.

Cooking Tip: Make your own whole-grain bread crumbs using stale bread or ends. Toast the bread, cut or break it into pieces, and crumble the toast pieces in the blender or food processor. Store in a jar in the refrigerator or freezer.

Note: Green beans can be substituted for the asparagus.

Nutritional Stars: Vitamin A, vitamin B3, vitamin E, folic acid

 # Grilled Vegetable Lasagna

Yield: 8 to 12 servings   100% vegetarian

This recipe requires you to puree cooked beans until they are a little soupy, a step that you can perform up to two days in advance. You'll save time but not lose flavor by using uncooked noodles, which absorb the liquids and flavors while the lasagna is baking.

PMS Benefits: To get the most out of your PMS diet, start with quality ingredients and then choose a cooking technique that preserves the vitamins and minerals. Instead of boiling vegetables in water, quick-grill them. In this lasagna, the baked vegetables release their nutrient-rich juices, which comingle with the delicious sauce!

Before you begin, soak 1 cup sorted and washed dried Great Northern or navy beans in 5 cups purified water for 6 hours or overnight.

> 2 **cups soaked Great Northern or navy beans (from 1 cup dried beans)**
> 5 **cups purified water**
> 1 **bay leaf**
> 2 **tablespoons extra-virgin olive oil**
> 1 **tablespoon balsamic or cider vinegar**
> ½ **teaspoon dried basil**
> ½ **teaspoon dried oregano**
> ¼ **teaspoon sea salt plus additional as needed**
>   **Ground black pepper**
> 2 **small yellow summer squash or zucchini, ends trimmed**

1 **eggplant, ends trimmed**
2 **red bell peppers, seeded**
2 **tablespoons unsalted butter, preferably organic, or additional extra-
   virgin olive oil**
2 **onions, sliced**
2 **cloves garlic, minced**
1 **teaspoon herbal sea salt**
¼ **teaspoon ground white pepper**
1 **recipe Chunky Onion-Celery Tomato Sauce (see page 203 and Note)**
2 **8-ounce boxes whole wheat lasagna noodles**
½ **cup grated pecorino Romano or Parmesan cheese, preferably
   organic (optional)**
8 **ounces mozzarella, preferably organic, grated (optional)**

1. With your hands or a slotted spoon, remove the beans from the soaking water to a large pot with the water and bay leaf. Bring to a boil, covered, lower heat, and simmer until tender, about 45 minutes.

2. Position the broiler shelf about 3 inches from the heat source. Preheat the broiler or preheat a grill.

3. In a wide bowl, mix together the olive oil, balsamic or cider vinegar, basil, oregano, ¼ teaspoon salt, and a pinch of black pepper.

4. Cut both the summer squash or zucchini and the eggplant lengthwise and then into ¼- to ½-inch slices. Cut the red peppers into quarters. Dip the vegetable slices into the herb mixture and place on a baking sheet; broil until lightly golden, 2 to 3 minutes. Using a fork or tongs, turn the vegetables over and broil on the other side. The vegetables do not need to be fully cooked.

5. In a sauté pan, heat the butter or olive oil and add the onions and garlic. Cook on medium-high heat for 2 minutes. Season with 2 pinches each of sea salt and black pepper. Cover and cook on medium heat for 10 minutes. Stir occasionally.

6. Place a colander in a bowl and pour in the beans. In a blender or food processor, puree the beans with half the cooking liquid. (Save the remaining cooking liquid for soup or use as stock.) Stir in the herbal sea salt and white pepper. The bean puree should be a little thin, and more liquid can be added, if needed.

7. Pour the pureed beans into the sauté pan with the onions and garlic. Stir well.

8. Position the oven shelves for the lasagna pan to fit into the middle of the oven. Preheat the oven to 350 degrees.

9. Prepare a deep baking pan with a generous layer of sauce, covering the entire bottom of the pan. Place a layer of uncooked lasagna noodles on top of the sauce. Pour 1 to 1½ cups sauce over the pasta and spread it evenly. Arrange all of the eggplant slices in a layer on top of the sauce. Spread one-third of the bean puree on top of the eggplant. Repeat with another layer of pasta, and spread over more

(Grilled Vegetable Lasagna—Continued)

sauce. Place the red peppers in a single layer and then another one-third of the bean puree. Follow this with a second layer of pasta and sauce, the summer squash or zucchini, and top with the remaining bean puree. Lastly, cover the lasagna with a remaining layer of noodles. Pour over more sauce in a thick layer and top with the grated Romano or Parmesan cheese and mozzarella, if using.

10. Cover the lasagna with parchment paper and foil, place in the oven, and bake for 45 minutes. Remove the parchment paper and foil and continue baking for another 10 to 15 minutes to allow the top to brown.

11. Remove the lasagna from the oven and allow it to cool and settle, about 10 minutes. Keep loosely covered with the parchment paper and foil.

12. Cut into 12 large pieces and serve with salad.

Cooking Tip: Cooking in, and covering foods with, parchment paper is far preferable to cooking in or on aluminum foil, especially if ingredients include acidic foods such as tomatoes. Exposed to acid, aluminum can leach from the foil and deposit in the food.

Note: If you prefer to use bottled tomato sauce, 1½ to 2 bottles will be needed. Dilute these with 1½ to 2 cups purified water. See the Appendix for suggested sugar-free brands.

Nutritional Stars: Vitamin A, B-complex vitamins, iron, manganese, zinc

From the Sea

Easy Fish Dishes

Delicious Shellfish Morsels

Fresh Seafood Benefits

A must-have staple of your PMS diet, fish—freshwater, saltwater, and shellfish—provides minerals including calcium, magnesium, iron, and zinc, which treat a range of PMS symptoms, from fatigue and breast tenderness to feeling blue and out of sorts. Seafood also supplies potassium and phosphorous, which are essential for general good health, as well as the fat-soluble vitamins A and D. While the fat content of fish and shellfish changes depending on the season and species, fatty fish such as salmon, mackerel, and halibut are good sources of these vitamins throughout the year. Vitamin A reduces fluid retention and uncomfortable menstrual bloating. All these minerals and vitamins are important in an overall nutrition program for PMS.

Fish also contains essential fatty acids, specifically the omega-3's, which are abundant in the sex glands and many of the other most biochemically active tissues in the body. The omega-3's convert to hormonelike compounds that ease menstrual cramping and lower back pain that many women experience once menstruation has begun. High amounts of these omega-3 fatty acids are found in the meatier fish from cold waters, such as salmon, herring, and sardines. For example, four ounces of salmon yields up to 3,600 milligrams of omega-3 fatty acids, while the same amount of cod (a low-fat fish) contains only 300 milligrams.

Excellent sources of easy-to-digest protein, fish and shellfish have more protein, less fat, and fewer calories per serving than most meat. An added bonus is the deliciously mild and light taste of fresh fish, an easy-to-like food if your menstrual symptoms include a queasy stomach that demands lighter dishes.

Although you may be concerned about polluted waters contaminating our fish supply, we believe it's safe to eat seafood regularly if you eat a variety of fish and shellfish, and have these no more than a maximum of two or three times a week.

Purchasing and Storing Fresh Fish

When purchasing fresh, whole fish, look for bright, clear, and bulging eyes; glossy skin, tight scales; and flesh that is firm when gently pressed. The fish store should have a fresh and clean ocean smell and no residual odor of ammonia, iodine, or "fishiness." Buy fish from markets that keep fish in chipped ice, not packaged in plastic.

When choosing prepared fillets, look for luminous and translucent pieces, firm to the touch. The fillet should not look flaky, dry, or dull, and should be displayed covered in ice chips. For the freshest-tasting fish, buy whole fish and have it filleted while waiting.

To ensure your fish maintains its freshness, buy and use the fish the same day. Make the fish store your last place to shop and then refrigerate the fish in the coldest part of the refrigerator. If your journey home is far, pack the fish in ice to keep it fresh.

There is no substitute for the taste of fresh fish and shellfish on your PMS diet, and we encourage you to add this to your shopping list—or to order fresh baked or broiled fish when you eat out.

 ## Fast Salmon with Lemon, Garlic, and Capers

Yield: 4 servings

Squeeze on lemon juice and add garlic and capers to any fish and it will be superb! Our favorite is salmon, but halibut, haddock, and tuna are equally delicious. Try some wild salmon—it is especially rich in omega-3 fatty acids.

PMS Benefits: To treat your symptoms of PMS, choose fish over red meat. Fish contains healthy amounts of omega-3 fatty acids, which combat menstrual cramping and discomfort. These important fats can be found in most cold-water fish, such as mackerel, tuna, and bluefish.

> 4 **tablespoons unsalted butter, preferably organic**
> 4 **½-inch salmon steaks, 1 to 1½ pounds**
> 2 **cloves garlic, slivered**
> ½ **teaspoon dried marjoram or thyme**
>   **Sea salt**
>   **Ground pepper**
> 2 **teaspoons capers**
> 1 **lemon, cut in half**

1. In a large sauté pan (big enough to fit all of the steaks at once), on medium heat, melt the butter.

2. Rinse the salmon under cold running water. Dry the steaks with paper toweling. Place them in the sauté pan and sprinkle with the garlic, marjoram or thyme, 2 pinches salt, and 1 pinch pepper. Cook on medium-high heat, uncovered, until the steaks begin to turn golden, 2 to 3 minutes.

3. Using a spatula, turn the steaks over and sprinkle the other side with 2 pinches salt, and 1 pinch pepper. Add the capers and squeeze the juice from half the lemon over the salmon. Cover and cook on a medium flame until the fish begins to flake and is tender when a fork is inserted, 10 to 12 minutes.

4. Remove the steaks to a serving platter. Cut the remaining lemon half into four wedges and place one wedge on top of each steak. Serve hot.

Cooking Tip: Capers are the flower bud that is picked, sun-dried, and either pickled in vinegar brine or packed in salt. They can be rinsed in water to remove excess salt.

Nutritional Stars: B-complex vitamins, vitamin B12, vitamin E, calcium, omega-3 fatty acids

 # Sun-drenched Grecian Red Snapper

Yield: 4 servings

A day on any Greek isle will stimulate a wave of hunger. We head for a beachside taverna and choose a fish from the kitchen for the chef to grill. We enjoy the flaky pieces with chunks of chewy bread dunked in a simple sauce of lemon and olive oil.

PMS Benefits: High in easy-to-digest protein, fish can help to lessen those symptoms of PMS that may include gastric upset.

Extra-virgin olive oil
4 **small or 2 large red snapper fillets, 1 to 1½ pounds (see Note)**
1 **lemon, cut in half**
2 **cloves garlic, minced**
1 **teaspoon dried oregano or marjoram**
¼ **teaspoon sea salt**
Several pinches ground pepper

1. Position the broiler shelf about 3 inches from the heat source. Preheat the broiler.

2. Drizzle a little olive oil on the bottom of a nonglass baking pan. Under cold running water, rinse the fillets. With paper toweling, pat them dry. Place the fillets in the baking pan.

3. Drizzle 1 or 2 teaspoons olive oil on each fillet. Squeeze half the lemon over the fillets and then sprinkle evenly with the garlic, oregano, salt, and pepper. Place under the broiler and cook until the fish begins to flake and is tender when a fork is inserted.

4. Cut the remaining lemon half into four pieces. Place the fish on a serving platter and serve with the lemon wedges.

Cooking Tip: Here's a quick way to test if your fish is completely cooked. When cooking a whole fish or fillets, insert a fork into the thickest section. The fork should slide in and out easily. Fillets will also begin to flake.

Note: Try flounder, monkfish, cod, or catfish instead of the red snapper.

Nutritional Stars: B-complex vitamins, omega-3 fatty acids

Tuna Steaks with Shallots and Apple Essence

Yield: 4 servings

A taste of apple juice lends a light sweetness to the tuna and the garlicky flavor of the shallots. A fish dish that is easy to prepare is worth making many times—as we know you will with this one.

PMS Benefits: Baking, broiling, poaching, or lightly sautéing fish and shellfish prevent their important fats and oils from overheating and turning toxic. Deep-frying, on the other hand, can turn these essential fats into *trans* fatty acids that can block the formation of certain prostaglandins, hormonelike compounds that lessen menstrual distress.

4 **tablespoons unsalted butter, preferably organic**
4 **shallots, sliced**
2 **cloves garlic, minced**
1 **1-inch piece fresh ginger, peeled and minced**
4 **½-inch halibut steaks, 1 to 1½ pounds**
   Sea salt
   Ground pepper
1 **cup unsweetened apple juice or ginger apple juice**
1 **bay leaf, broken in half**
1 **lemon, cut into wedges**
   Fresh mint or basil leaves for garnish

1. In a large skillet, on medium heat, melt the butter and sauté the shallots, garlic, and ginger until bubbling, about 2 minutes. Stir frequently.

2. Under cold running water, rinse the steaks. With paper toweling, pat them dry. Place the steaks on top of the shallot mixture and sprinkle each with 2 pinches salt and 1 pinch pepper. Cook on high heat for 1 minute to sear the outside. Using a spatula, carefully turn the steaks over and sear the other side for 1 minute. Sprinkle again with the salt and pepper.

3. Pour in the apple juice and add the bay leaf. Cover and on high heat bring the liquid to a boil. Lower the flame and simmer until the fish is tender when a fork is inserted, 7 to 10 minutes.

4. Remove the steaks to a platter, cover, and place in the oven to keep warm.

5. Bring the liquid in the skillet to a boil uncovered. Continue cooking until half of the pan juices have evaporated.

6. Remove the bay leaf. Spoon the juices over the steaks and serve with lemon wedges. Garnish with the mint or basil leaves.

Cooking Tip: The thickness of the fish will help you to determine the approximate cooking time. Estimate 7 to 10 minutes per ½-inch thickness.

Nutritional Stars: B-complex vitamins, vitamin B12, iron, omega-3 fatty acids

 # Portuguese Halibut with Red Pepper Slices and Green Olives

Yield: 4 servings

We had a version of this in a great restaurant called Restaurante Guaquin in Costa del Sol, Spain. We liked it so much we licked our plates clean. Try this fantastic sauce with grains, pasta, or beans.

PMS Benefits: Fish is a terrific source of minerals, including potassium, iodine, zinc, and copper, plus the omega-3 fatty acids, all of which are low in the diets of women with PMS—and most Americans. Halibut also contains vitamin B3, which helps us metabolize sugar and stabilize the cluster of menstrual symptoms related to carbohydrate cravings. Magnesium helps maintain the brain chemistry that regulates PMS emotions, and halibut also contains an ample amount of it.

  2 **tablespoons unsalted butter, preferably organic, or additional extra-virgin olive oil**
  2 **onions, sliced**
  2 **cloves garlic, sliced**
  2 **ripe tomatoes, cores removed, chopped**
  1 **red bell pepper, seeded and sliced**
  ¾ **teaspoon herbal sea salt**
  ¼ **teaspoon ground pepper**
  6 **teaspoons extra-virgin olive oil**
  1 **to 1½ pounds halibut fillet**
  1 **lemon, cut in half**
  ½ **cup pitted green olives or 2 tablespoons capers**
  ½ **cup homemade salt-free stock or purified water**

(Portuguese Halibut with Red Pepper Slices and Green Olives—Continued)

1. In a large skillet, heat the butter and add the onions, garlic, tomatoes, and red pepper. Sauté on a medium-high flame for 2 minutes. Stir frequently.

2. Sprinkle with ½ teaspoon herbal sea salt and ¼ teaspoon pepper and stir again. Cover and cook on medium-low heat for 10 minutes.

3. Position the broiler shelf about 3 inches from the heat source. Preheat the broiler.

4. Drizzle 1 teaspoon olive oil into a nonglass baking pan. Rinse the halibut under cold running water. With paper toweling, dry the fillets. Place the halibut in the baking pan and squeeze half the lemon all over. Season with the remaining 5 teaspoons olive oil, ¼ teaspoon herbal sea salt, and a pinch of pepper. Place under the broiler and cook until the fish begins to flake and is tender when a fork is inserted, 8 to 10 minutes.

5. Stir the tomato–red pepper mixture. Add the olives or capers and stock or water and stir well. Cook another 1 or 2 minutes, uncovered.

6. Using a large spatula, remove the cooked halibut to a large serving platter. Top with the red pepper and olive mixture. Cut the remaining half lemon into wedges and place on the platter. Serve while hot with cooked rice or potatoes.

Cooking Tip: Lemon juice and vinegar are good flavor enhancers and are often used in addition to salt. Their use lowers the amount of sodium needed in a recipe.

Nutritional Stars: Vitamin B3, vitamin B12, iron, magnesium, omega-3 fatty acids

Easy Trout Baked in a Light Mustard Sauce

Yield: 4 servings

Trout is a mild white-meat fish that cooks quickly. The bones are mostly around the belly and are relatively easy to remove. And remember to eat the skin, which contains the important essential fatty acids.

PMS Benefits: Do yourself a PMS favor and get into the habit of buying organic butter, which you'll find in natural-food stores or in supermarket chains that feature natural foods. Antibiotics and hormones routinely fed to some livestock accumulate in the fatty tissue of the animal. Ordinary butter is potentially a loaded source of these compounds that can upset your own hormone balance.

¼ **cup purified water**
2 **tablespoons prepared mustard**
2 **tablespoons extra-virgin olive oil or unsalted butter, preferably organic**
2 **cloves garlic, minced**
¼ **teaspoon sea salt**
   Pinch ground pepper
1 **to 1½ pounds trout, butterflied**

1. Position the oven shelves so that a baking pan fits in the center. Preheat the oven to 350 degrees.

2. In a small bowl, mix the water, mustard, olive oil or butter, garlic, salt, and pepper. Pour half into a baking pan large enough for the trout.

3. Under cold running water, rinse the trout. With paper toweling, dry the fish. Place the fish in the baking pan on top of the sauce and pour the remaining sauce over the fish. Cover with parchment and foil. Put the fish in the oven and bake until it begins to flake and the fish is tender when a fork is inserted, about 15 minutes.

4. Place on a warm platter and serve with a whole grain and a salad.

Cooking Tip: We recommend extra-virgin olive oil, which is produced from the first pressing of the olives and not refined in any way. Manufacturers both heat and add chemical solvents to virgin and pure olive oils, which changes their taste and beneficial nutrients.

Nutritional Stars: B-complex vitamins, vitamin B12, omega-3 fatty acids

 # Cod Cakes with Avocado Mayonnaise

Yield: 4 to 6 servings

Also referred to as "poor man's crab cakes." A fine way for fish to find its way onto the PMS menu—plus almost everyone will love them.

PMS Benefits: Add quality protein and minerals, lower the fat content in your diet, and treat your PMS symptoms with a fresh fish such as cod. The high fat content of beef, lamb, or pork may only aggravate your PMS problems.

(Cod Cakes with Avocado Mayonnaise—Continued)

The cod cakes:

1 pound cod, flounder, red snapper, or other white-meat fillet, cut
into chunks
1 egg, preferably organic
2 stalks celery, ends trimmed, minced
2 cloves garlic, minced
1 onion, minced
4 sprigs fresh parsley, washed, thick stems removed, and minced
¼ to ½ cup whole-grain bread crumbs
½ teaspoon herbal sea salt
¼ teaspoon ground pepper
½ teaspoon dried thyme or basil
¼ cup extra-virgin olive oil
¼ cup ghee (see page 227) or unsalted butter, preferably organic

The mayonnaise:

1 ripe avocado
1 tablespoon cider vinegar
1 teaspoon prepared mustard
¼ teaspoon sea salt
1 tablespoon purified water plus additional as needed
½ lemon, cut into wedges

The cod cakes:

1. In a blender or food processor, pulse-chop the cod. Place in a large bowl and add the egg, celery, garlic, onion, parsley, ¼ cup bread crumbs, herbal sea salt, pepper, and thyme or basil. Mix very well. Add more bread crumbs if needed to keep the mixture from crumbling.

2. In a large sauté pan, heat ¼ cup each of olive oil and ghee or unsalted butter.

3. Wet your hands lightly with water. Form the fish mixture into six to eight cakes, about ½ inch thick. Place them in the hot oil and cook until the underside is golden, 7 to 8 minutes. Using a spatula, carefully turn the cakes over and cook on the other side until golden, another 6 to 7 minutes. Remove to a brown bag or paper toweling to drain.

The mayonnaise:

1. Cut the avocado in half and remove the pit. Using a spoon, scoop the avocado flesh out of the skin and put it into a blender or food processor. Add the vinegar, mustard, salt, and water and puree until smooth. Add more water as needed to puree smoothly. (It should not be runny.)

2. Serve the Cod Cakes while hot with Avocado Mayonnaise on the side and the lemon wedges. Add a salad and a whole-grain roll for a complete meal.

Cooking Tip: To save yourself from mincing, pulse-mince to a fine consistency the celery, onions, garlic, and parsley in a food processor or a minichopper.

Nutritional Stars: Vitamin B5, vitamin B12

 # Sea Scallops with Salsa Cruda

Yield: 4 servings

These scallops are tossed with a raw-vegetable sauce, which is at room temperature when served. Pour the crunchy, cool vegetable sauce over a bed of hot scallops—the scallops cool down and the salsa heats up! We find this a perfect dish to serve in late summer or early fall. Make it ahead of time and refrigerate until about 10 minutes before serving.

PMS Benefits: A good source of low-fat protein, shellfish also supplies trace minerals such as iodine, fluorine, and cobalt. It is important to consume all the nutrients of a healthful diet, including these valuable trace minerals, to support the intricate chemistry of your body both before and after menstruation.

The scallops:

- 1 to 1½ pounds sea scallops (see Note)
- ¼ cup unsalted butter, preferably organic, or extra-virgin olive oil
- 2 cloves garlic, minced
- 4 sprigs fresh parsley, washed, thick stems removed, and minced
- ½ teaspoon herbal sea salt
- ¼ teaspoon ground pepper
   Juice of 1 lemon

The salsa:

- 2 cloves garlic, minced
- 1 red onion, minced

(Sea Scallops with Salsa Cruda—Continued)

    2 ripe tomatoes, cores removed, chopped fine
      Juice of 1 lime (3 tablespoons)
  ½ bunch fresh cilantro (coriander), washed, thick stems
      removed, and minced
    4 sprigs fresh dill, washed, thick stems removed, minced
    3 tablespoons extra-virgin olive oil
    1 tablespoon flaxseed oil

The scallops:

1. Fill a bowl with cold water and add the scallops. Place a colander in the sink and remove the scallops to drain. Put several paper towels on a work surface and place the scallops on them to dry, using one or two towels to pat the tops dry.

2. In a large skillet, heat the butter or oil. Add the garlic and parsley and cook until they begin to bubble, about 1 minute. Stir frequently.

3. Add the scallops and sear them in the hot pan for 1 minute. Turn and sear the other side, cooking for another minute.

4. Add the herbal sea salt, pepper, and lemon juice. Cover and steam on medium heat until the scallops are tender when a fork is inserted, 7 to 10 minutes. Do not overcook or they will become rubbery.

The salsa:

1. In a medium-sized bowl, stir together the garlic, red onion, tomatoes, lime juice, cilantro, dill, and the oils.

2. Place the cooked scallops on a platter and top with the Salsa Cruda. Serve immediately.

Cooking Tip: For this dish we prefer sea scallops because their flavor is superior to that of bay scallops. The texture of the sea scallops is tender and almost creamy when cooked to perfection, as recommended.

Note: Bay scallops can be substituted if sea scallops are not available. Reduce the cooking time in Step 4 to 3 or 4 minutes.

Nutritional Stars: Copper, iodine, magnesium, zinc

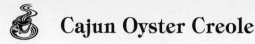 # Cajun Oyster Creole

Yield: 4 servings

Take a quick trip to Louisiana when you dig into this abundant and nutrient-rich stew.

PMS Benefits: Shellfish such as shrimp, crab, and oysters are a great source of vitamins and minerals that can put the brakes on PMS. A remarkable answer to your SOS for PMS, oysters contain a sunken treasure of nutrients—B-complex, vitamins C and E, folic acid, calcium, copper, iron, magnesium, zinc, and omega-3 fatty acids, all of which are on the PMS menu. Try this recipe if you're feeling peevish, weighted down, or out of sorts.

   4 **tablespoons extra-virgin olive oil or unsalted butter, preferably organic**
   4 **beefsteak or 8 plum tomatoes, cores removed, chopped**
   1 **red bell pepper, seeded and diced**
   1 **green bell pepper, seeded and diced**
   1 **onion, sliced**
   2 **cloves garlic, minced**
   1 **bay leaf**
   ¼ **teaspoon ground black pepper plus additional as needed**
   ¼ **teaspoon ground white pepper**
      Pinch red pepper flakes
   1 **teaspoon herbal sea salt**
   2 **pints shucked oysters and juice (approximately 3 dozen)**
      Cider or brown rice vinegar
      Hot sauce

1. In a large sauté pan, heat 2 tablespoons olive oil or butter and add the tomatoes, red and green peppers, onion, garlic, and bay leaf. Season with black, white, and red pepper, and ½ teaspoon herbal sea salt. Cover and cook on medium-low heat for 15 minutes. Stir occasionally.

2. Place a fine mesh sieve or cheesecloth-lined colander over a bowl. Pour in the oysters and liquid. Remove the oysters from the sieve into a medium-sized bowl, as the liquid is draining. Reserve the liquid. Inspect the oysters for any remaining shell fragments.

3. Under cold running water, rinse the oysters, rubbing lightly to loosen grit and sand. Place in a separate colander to drain.

4. Place the oysters on top of the vegetable mixture. Drizzle with 2 tablespoons olive oil, ½ teaspoon herbal sea salt, a pinch black pepper, and a splash of vinegar. Cover and cook until the oysters are tender when a fork is inserted, 5 to 7 minutes.

(Cajun Oyster Creole—Continued)

5. Remove bay leaf. Using a large spatula, remove the Cajun Oyster Creole to a serving platter. Serve immediately with a bottle of hot sauce on the side.

Cooking Tip: The use of salt is a matter of personal preference and tolerance. We usually prefer to add only a small amount of salt. If you are someone who has cut back on salt intake, you'll find our recipes just about right for your taste. If you want more, add another dash.

Nutritional Stars: B-complex vitamins, vitamin C, vitamin E, folic acid, calcium, copper, iron, magnesium, zinc, omega-3 fatty acids

 ## Clam and Shrimp Bouillabaisse

Yield: 4 servings

This soupy shellfish stew is easy to make and a tasty way to add seafood to the PMS menu. Pick up your clams and shrimp just hours before dinnertime to enjoy a really fresh taste and the beneficial nutrients seafood can offer.

PMS Benefits: Some people avoid shellfish in fear of the cholesterol it contains, but some shellfish, such as scallops and crab, contain no more cholesterol than the dark meat in chicken. We give a green light to gently cooked shellfish and applaud its many minerals that soothe menstrual inflammation and moody irritation!

Before you begin, prepare the shrimp stock. Follow the directions in Step 1.

- 12 to 16 uncooked jumbo shrimp with shells
- 3 cups purified water
- 1 bay leaf
- 1 teaspoon cider vinegar
- 4 tablespoons extra-virgin olive oil
- 4 ripe beefsteak tomatoes or 10 plum tomatoes, cores removed, chopped
- 1 onion, minced
- 4 cloves garlic, sliced
- 1 teaspoon herbal sea salt
- ¼ teaspoon ground pepper
  Pinch red pepper flakes or ½ teaspoon hot sauce
- 12 to 16 fresh clams, shells washed
- ½ pound sea scallops

½ **pound white-meat fish, such as haddock, flounder, catfish, or fluke**
2 **tablespoons unsalted butter, preferably organic**
4 **to 6 sprigs fresh parsley, washed, thick stems removed, and minced coarsely**

1. Remove the shells from the shrimp and set the shrimp aside. Put the shells into a medium-sized saucepan with the water, bay leaf, and vinegar. Bring to a boil, covered. Reduce the heat to medium, leave the lid partly uncovered, and simmer until the stock reduces to 2 cups, about 30 minutes.

2. Devein the shrimp and wash in cold water. Refrigerate until ready to use.

3. In a large soup pot or Dutch oven, heat 2 tablespoons olive oil and add the tomatoes, onion, and garlic. Cover and cook on a medium flame for 10 minutes. Stir occasionally.

4. Hold a fine-meshed strainer over the tomato mixture, and pour the shrimp stock through it. Discard the shells and bay leaf. Stir well and bring to a boil, covered.

5. Season the tomato broth with the herbal sea salt, pepper, and pepper flakes or hot sauce. Add the shrimp and clams, and return to a boil, covered. Cook 1 minute.

6. Add the scallops and fish. Spoon some of the tomato broth over the fish and add the remaining 2 tablespoons olive oil and the butter. Cook covered, on medium heat, until the fish begins to flake, about 2 minutes.

7. Pour the bouillabaisse into a large serving bowl and top with the parsley. Serve with garlic bruschetta or brown rice.

Cooking Tip: Seafood is highly perishable and is best used within hours of purchase. During the warmer months, have a bag of ice packed in with the fish to keep it cool while transporting it home.

Nutritional Stars: Vitamin B2, vitamin B3, vitamin B12, vitamin E, calcium, copper, iron, magnesium

From the Land

Poultry

Beef

Pork

Lamb

Nutrient Benefits of Poultry and Meat

Though the PMS diet tends to emphasize protein-rich vegetables and seafood over red meat, have no fear if you're a meat lover because poultry and meat still have many benefits to offer. These foods are rich in B-complex vitamins that work together with a variety of minerals to treat the symptoms of PMS. For instance, treat the anemia that results from heavy menstrual bleeding with the replenishing iron found in meat. Steaks and chops will also give you long-lasting energy to combat the fatigue many women feel toward the end of their menstrual cycles.

The quality of the meat you eat is vital to your menstrual health. Cook with organic or free-range poultry and meats that do not contain added hormones and antibiotics. Unlike commercially raised animals, free-range breeds grow in more natural conditions with sunlight and exercise, and they are much lower in fat. Such foods are more widely available than ever before. (See the Appendix for sources.) Yes, meats and poultry without the added chemicals are a little more expensive, but we think they're worth it.

Research shows that women who consume lower amounts of animal fat experience less menstrual bloating, breast tenderness, and weight gain. If you are sensitive to the fats in meat, switch to low-fat white-meat chicken and turkey.

Depending on how you feel each month, you may comfortably tolerate meat and poultry once in a while. Choose a lean cut, and have a small portion of about 3 to 4 ounces. This amounts to a hamburger patty the size of the palm of your hand—not very large by American standards.

Purchasing and Handling Meats

There are two ways in which meat quality is regulated in the marketplace. The U.S. Department of Agriculture inspects all meats sold interstate. (Locally butchered meats, however, are not subject to these same regulations.) The U.S. government also regulates meats packaged and sold by wholesale companies, which are graded according to federal standards for juiciness, flavor, and tenderness. Free-range and organically raised animals are inspected using these same national standards.

When buying meat, allow ¼ pound per serving for the trimmed and boneless cuts, which includes flank, tenderloin, steaks, and boned roasts. If the bone is left in, allow ⅓ pound per serving, as in the case of rib roasts, bone-in steaks, chops, and ham roasts.

Store meat and poultry in the coldest part of the refrigerator. Ground meat is the most perishable and should be used within twenty-four hours of purchase. Cubed and diced meat is best used within forty-eight hours, while steaks will keep for two to four days, and roasts three to four days. Also, note that pork, lamb, and veal are slightly more perishable than beef, and poultry is the most perishable of all and should be kept well refrigerated until preparation time.

When freezing, first wrap your meat and poultry in freezer paper. Avoid using plastic wrap, which is semipermeable and allows moisture to evaporate causing freezer burn. To defrost meat and poultry, place them on a plate or in a baking pan and thaw in the refrigerator. Depending on the size, thawing time takes two to four days. Before you cook, make sure your cuts of meat are completely defrosted to ensure thorough cooking. Use a meat thermometer inserted into the densest area of the meat away from the bone. For safety's sake, consume cooked meat and poultry within five days. To preserve a stuffed and cooked bird, remove the stuffing from its cavity before refrigerating the meat, and chill the stuffing in a separate container.

 # Roasted Chicken with Kasha and Wild Mushroom Stuffing

Yield: 4 servings

This is a whole meal in one recipe—just add a salad. Use any leftover chicken to make a tasty sandwich for lunch or a quick and easy chicken salad.

PMS Benefits: Skinless poultry contains lower levels of fat than most cuts of red meat. Research shows that animal fats stimulate the growth of the intestinal bacteria that reabsorb estrogen about to be excreted. This can lead to elevated levels of estrogen in circulation and symptoms of anxiety associated with this imbalance. Building meals around leaner meats such as white-meat chicken prevents excessive estrogen accumulation.

The chicken:

1   2½- to 3-pound chicken, preferably organic
1   lemon, preferably organic
    Sea salt
    Sage or rosemary
    Ground pepper

The stuffing:

2   cups purified water or homemade salt-free stock
1   cup kasha or quinoa
1   teaspoon herbal sea salt

 8 **ounces mixed wild mushrooms, such as portobello, cremini,**
   and oyster
 2 **tablespoons unsalted butter, preferably organic, or extra-virgin olive oil**
 2 **onions, minced**
 2 **cloves garlic, minced**
 2 **teaspoons fennel seeds**
 1 **apple, preferably organic, core removed, grated or chopped**
 ½ **cup unsulphured currants**
 ½ **cup raw walnuts, chopped coarsely**

Position the oven shelves so that the baking pan fits in the center. Preheat the oven to 350 degrees.

The chicken:

1. Under cold running water, wash the chicken cavity. With paper toweling, pat the chicken dry and put it into a baking pan, breast side up.

2. Squeeze the lemon over all the chicken and then put the squeezed halves into the cavity. Sprinkle the chicken and the cavity with salt, sage or rosemary, and pepper.

3. Put the chicken in the preheated oven, uncovered. Roast until the leg juices run clear when pricked with a fork, 45 to 55 minutes. Turn the chicken over halfway through cooking.

The stuffing:

1. In a saucepan, bring the water or stock to a boil, covered. Add the kasha or quinoa and ½ teaspoon herbal sea salt. Return to a boil, reduce flame, and simmer until the liquid is absorbed, about 10 minutes.

2. Wash the mushrooms and chop coarsely. Heat the butter or olive oil in an oven-proof sauté pan. Add the mushrooms with the onions, garlic, and fennel seeds. Cover and cook until the onions become translucent, about 10 minutes. Stir occasionally.

3. Add the apple, currants, walnuts, and ½ teaspoon herbal sea salt. Stir well. Cover and cook 5 more minutes.

4. Using a large fork, scratch the surface of the cooked grain to fluff and separate the grains. Mix into the onion mixture, combining well.

5. Place the sauté pan in the oven and cook until the top browns slightly and the nuts start to roast, 20 to 30 minutes. Stir occasionally.

Cooking Tip: To save time and mess, we cook the stuffing separately. This ensures that the interior of the chicken will be properly cooked.

Nutritional Stars: Vitamin B3, vitamin B5, vitamin B6, folic acid, flavonoids, zinc

Curried Chicken and Vegetable Stir-fry

Yield: 4 servings

Stir-frying is an ancient quick-cooking technique and is still a great way to save time and energy in the kitchen. Before you run out of steam at the end of the day, simply toss these flavorful ingredients together and refuel yourself.

PMS Benefits: Poultry is a good source of versatile, low-fat protein. It contains the B-complex vitamins, especially niacin (B3), and the minerals iron and phosphorus. White meat is higher in niacin, while dark is especially high in thiamin (B1) and riboflavin (B2). Eat some of both to prevent PMS mood swings and depression.

4 **boneless chicken cutlets, preferably organic**
2 **tablespoons ghee (see page 227) or extra-virgin olive oil**
2 **onions, sliced**
3 **cloves garlic, sliced**
1 **tablespoon curry powder**
1 **1-inch piece ginger, grated or minced**
1 **green bell pepper, seeded and sliced thin**
1 **red bell pepper, seeded and sliced thin**
2 **stalks celery, ends trimmed, sliced**
1 **teaspoon sea salt**
1½ **cups homemade salt-free stock or purified water**
1 **tablespoon arrowroot or kuzu powder (see page 228)**
2 **tablespoons dark sesame oil**

1. Cut the chicken cutlets into thin strips. Set aside.

2. In a wok or large sauté pan, heat the ghee or olive oil and add the onions and garlic. Cook on medium-high heat until the onion edges begin to brown, about 10 minutes. Stir occasionally.

3. Add the curry powder and ginger, and stir. Cook for 30 seconds. Add the green and red peppers, celery, and salt. Lower heat and cook covered, until the peppers begin to soften, 2 or 3 minutes.

4. Add the chicken and 1 cup stock or water. Cover and steam for 5 to 7 minutes.

5. Pour the remaining ½ cup stock or water into a small bowl containing the arrowroot or kuzu. Stir until dissolved. Make a well in the center of the pan (push the vegetables and chicken to the side) and pour the stock mixture in. Stir until the liquid begins to clear. Mix the thickening liquid through the vegetables and chicken and cook another 30 seconds. It will have a slightly glossy sheen.

6. Pour the dark sesame oil over the mixture and stir one last time. Serve with a bowl of brown rice or whole-grain noodles.

Cooking Tip: Dark sesame oil is made from roasted sesame seeds. Since the seeds have already been cooked and their flavor intensified, we prefer to add the oil at the end of the recipe as a flavoring.

Nutritional Stars: B-complex vitamins, vitamin C, zinc

 # Easy Roman Chicken Cutlet Parmesan

Yield: 4 to 6 servings

This is the lazy woman's way to prepare chicken cutlet Parmesan—no frying, less clean-up, and less fat. Your kitchen—and hips—will show it!

PMS Benefits: Poultry is a good source of vitamin A and the B-complex vitamins. Both of these nutrients play a role in reducing fatigue, one of the symptoms associated with carbohydrate cravings that many women experience each month. Lower in saturated fat than red meats, poultry is an excellent source of protein.

- 3 cups Chunky Onion-Celery Tomato Sauce (see page 203)
- 6 boneless chicken cutlets, preferably organic (see Note)
- ½ cup whole-grain bread crumbs
- 2 tablespoons grated Parmesan cheese
- 4 sprigs fresh parsley, washed, thick stems removed, and minced
- 2 tablespoons extra-virgin olive oil
- 2 cloves garlic, minced
- ½ teaspoon herbal sea salt
- ¼ teaspoon ground pepper
- 8 ounces mozzarella, preferably organic, cut into thin slices or grated

1. Position the oven shelves so that a baking pan fits in the center. Preheat the oven to 350 degrees.

2. In a blender or food processor, puree some or all of the sauce. Spread 1 cup of the sauce on the bottom of a deep baking pan.

3. Under cold running water, wash the cutlets. Pat them dry with paper toweling, and put them in the sauce in the baking pan.

4. In a small bowl, mix the bread crumbs, Parmesan cheese, parsley, olive oil,

(Easy Roman Chicken Cutlet Parmesan—Continued)

garlic, herbal sea salt, and pepper. Sprinkle the crumb mixture evenly over the cutlets. Cover each cutlet with the remaining 1 cup of sauce.

5. Place the mozzarella slices on top and cover with parchment paper and foil. Place in the oven and bake until the cutlets are tender, about 30 minutes.

6. Remove the parchment and foil, and continue baking until the cutlets are tender and the juices run clear when pricked with a fork, another 10 minutes.

7. In a small saucepan, heat the remaining ½ to 1 cup sauce. Using a spatula, remove the cutlets to a serving platter. Place the remaining sauce on the side with a serving spoon. Serve with a salad and whole-grain pasta for an enjoyable and filling meal.

Cooking Tip: To speed up the browning of a dish (in this case the mozzarella), place it under the broiler for 2 or 3 minutes. Make sure the pan is not glass, or the heat of the broiler will shatter it.

Note: The cutlets can be pounded to a ¼-inch thickness, or left as is.

Nutritional Stars: Vitamin A, B-complex vitamins, zinc

 Turkey for Two

Yield: 2 servings

Here's a simple recipe with a delicious taste that will satisfy your turkey cravings between the holidays. PS: It's easy to double this recipe.

PMS Benefits: Vitamin B6 is important for women with PMS because it alleviates symptoms such as headaches, bloating, depression, irritability, and fatigue. Poultry, including turkey, contains plentiful amounts of vitamin B6. Other sources are whole grains and many beans, nuts, and seeds.

    2 tablespoons unsalted butter, preferably organic, or extra-virgin olive oil
    1 turkey leg, preferably organic
    ½ lemon with rind, preferably organic
    ½ cup homemade salt-free stock or purified water
    ½ teaspoon dried sage
      Several pinches herbal sea salt
      Pinch ground pepper

1. In a medium-sized sauté pan, on high heat, heat the butter or olive oil. Add the turkey leg and brown on all sides. Use tongs to turn the leg as each side browns.

2. Squeeze the lemon juice all over. Cut the rind in half and add with the stock or water, sage, herbal sea salt, and pepper. Cover and cook on medium-low heat until tender when pierced with a fork, about 45 minutes.

3. Place the cooked turkey leg on a serving platter. Carve some of the meat off the bone and drizzle the pan juices over. Serve hot or at room temperature.

Cooking Tip: When a recipe calls for the skin of a lemon (or orange) we opt for organic—free from the pesticides and preservatives sprayed on the exterior of most citrus fruit.

Nutritional Stars: Vitamin B3, vitamin B6, folic acid, zinc

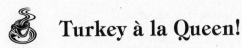

Turkey à la Queen!

Yield: 4 servings

Turkey is a low-fat bird with plenty of helpful PMS nutrients that can be cooked and enjoyed all year round, not just on holidays! After you've had your fill, make the leftovers into soup or a yummy stew.

PMS Benefits: Organic and free-range poultry is raised without the use of added hormones or antibiotics, compounds that can aggravate PMS symptoms in some women.

¼ **cup ghee (see page 227) or unsalted butter, preferably organic**
¼ **cup whole wheat flour**
2 **to 3 cups homemade salt-free stock or purified water**
1 **onion, chopped**
1 **carrot, ends trimmed, chopped**
½ **teaspoon sea salt**
    Pinch pepper
2 **cups leftover cooked turkey, preferably organic, diced or shredded**
½ **cup fresh peas or sugar snaps**

1. In a medium-sized sauté pan on moderate heat, melt the ghee or butter and stir in the flour. Cook until the flour begins to smell roasted and turns slightly golden brown, 5 to 7 minutes. Stir constantly, being careful not to burn.

2. Using a whisk, add the stock or water in ¼-cup amounts until the first cup has been incorporated. Stir well, allowing the mixture to reheat after each addition.

(Turkey à la Queen!—Continued)

Proceed by adding ½-cup amounts of the stock until enough additional stock has been added to make a thin sauce.

3. Stir the onion, carrot, salt, and pepper into the sauce. Cover and cook on medium heat until the vegetables soften, about 10 minutes.

4. Add the cooked turkey and peas or sugar snaps. Stir well, cover, and cook another 2 minutes.

5. Serve the creamy turkey over whole-grain English muffins, cooked noodles, or brown rice.

Cooking Tip: If there isn't any leftover cooked turkey available, bake either a boneless turkey or chicken breasts and cook them in the sauce before you add the vegetables. Begin at step 3.

Nutritional Stars: Vitamin A, vitamin B3, vitamin B6, folic acid, zinc

 # French Bistro Entrecôte

Yield: 4 servings

Plain and simple—beefsteak, as it's known in some parts, at its best. Easy to prepare at home, but with the taste of dinner in a French Bistro.

PMS Benefits: For some women, meat can cause many PMS symptoms. If you aren't as sensitive, try eating organic meats to avoid any further problems associated with the synthetic estrogens fed to some animals.

2 tablespoons unsalted butter, preferably organic
2 cloves garlic, chopped
4 small or 2 large beefsteaks, ¾ to 1 inch thick (about 1½ pounds),
**   preferably organic (see Note)**
4 teaspoons prepared mustard
**   Sea salt**
**   Freshly ground pepper**
½ cup homemade salt-free stock or purified water

1. In one or two large sauté pans (to fit all the steaks at once), melt the butter on high heat. Swirl the pans to coat the bottoms evenly. Add the garlic and stir once.

2. Lay the steaks in the pans in one layer, with ¼ to ½ inch between each. Spread a teaspoon of mustard on each steak. Sauté 1½ minutes. Using tongs or a large fork, turn the steaks over and sauté another 1½ minutes on the other side.

3. Season with the salt and pepper. Remove to individual hot plates or a hot platter. Quickly add the stock or water to the pan to deglaze the juices and flavors. Drizzle over the steaks. *Bon Appétit!*

Cooking Tip: It is somewhat of an art to test a steak without cutting it open. Press the steak with your finger and look for:
Red-rare—barely springy to the touch (not as soft as when raw)
Medium-rare—a little red juice on the surface
Well-done—no red juices appear on the surface
Note: Substitute T-bone, sirloin, top loin, porterhouse, tenderloin, rib eye, or any other favorite cut of beef.
Nutritional Stars: Vitamin B3, vitamin B6, folic acid, iron, zinc

 ## Strip Steak Pizzaiola

Yield: 4 servings

This recipe for steak is inspired by similar preparations we've had in Europe. Start with smaller cuts of meat and use some prepared or ready-made tomato sauce. Quick to cook, this pizzaiola is an easy meal when you are on overload. Bon Appétit!

PMS Benefits: Choose small cuts of lean meat to satisfy your craving. Three to four ounces, the equivalent of the size of the palm of your hand, will give you beneficial protein, as well as an ample serving of niacin, a vitamin essential for carbohydrate metabolism. Niacin helps ensure even blood-sugar levels and steady moods.

1   **recipe Chunky Onion-Celery Tomato Sauce (see page 203) or 2 cups prepared tomato sauce**
4   **strip or cube steaks, 1 to 1½ pounds, preferably organic**
    Sea salt
    Freshly ground pepper

1. Preheat a cast-iron grill, outdoor grill, or the broiler.
2. In a small saucepan on low heat, warm the sauce, covered.
3. Place the steaks on the grill surface (if using a broiler, place them on the

(Strip Steak Pizzaiola—Continued)

broiler pan) and cook about 1½ minutes to sear and lock in the juices. Turn the steaks over and cook to your preference, about another 1½ minutes.

4. Season with salt and pepper, and remove to individual hot plates or a hot platter. Ladle a thin layer of sauce over the steaks and serve right away.

Cooking Tip: Strip or cube steaks cook very quickly, so be careful not to overcook or they will become tough.

Nutritional Stars: Vitamin B3, vitamin B6, folic acid, flavonoids, iron, zinc

 ## Country-style Pork Spareribs Simmered in Barbecue Sauce

Yield: 4 servings

Here's a healthy way to delight in the taste of an outdoor barbecue without the added sugars in a store-bought sauce. If you're feeling southern, serve these tangy ribs alongside corn bread and slaw, and enjoy the healthful benefits of good food.

PMS Benefits: Red meats contain a wide variety of vitamins and minerals. Included in these are many of the B-complex vitamins, folic acid, and iron. Meat such as the pork in this recipe provides iron which can correct anemia that may be brought on by a heavy menstrual cycle.

Before you begin, prepare the barbecue sauce and marinate the ribs for 30 minutes or overnight.

 1 **cup Enrico's Mesquite Flavor Barbecue Sauce, tomato paste, or**
    sugar-free ketchup
 1 **onion, minced**
 4 **cloves garlic, minced**
 ½ **cup cider vinegar**
 ¼ **cup unsulphured blackstrap molasses**
 2 **tablespoons hot sauce (optional)**
 1 **teaspoon dried oregano**
 ½ **teaspoon sea salt**
 ¼ **teaspoon cayenne pepper**
 4 **to 6 country-style pork spareribs or bone-in pork chops, about**
    2 pounds, preferably organic

1. In a large bowl, mix the barbecue sauce, tomato paste, or ketchup with the onion, garlic, vinegar, molasses, hot sauce, oregano, salt, and cayenne. Add the spareribs, cover, and put in the refrigerator to marinate for at least 30 minutes or overnight.

2. Put the pork in one layer in a large skillet, and add all of the sauce. Bring to a boil, covered, on high heat. Lower flame and cook until the pork is tender when a fork is inserted, 40 to 50 minutes.

3. Serve with fingerling or mashed potatoes and a gorgeous green salad.

Cooking Tip: To peel garlic easily, use a "miracle garlic peeler"—it's a tube of soft and pliable rubber. Put the unpeeled cloves of garlic inside the tube and roll them back and forth. The skins come off and the garlic drops out peeled.

Nutritional Stars: Vitamin B6, vitamin B12, folic acid, iron

 # Garlic-roasted Fresh Ham

Yield: 6 to 8 servings

This is a terrific dish to prepare after the holidays. Have your butcher cut a fresh ham in two and store half in the freezer for future dinners. Even with half a ham, you will need a crowd to enjoy this finger-licking dish—and you'll still have left-overs for sandwiches during the week.

PMS Benefits: Many kitchen seasonings have medicinal properties that can ease PMS. The garlic in the recipe can treat acne by restoring alkalinity to the blood. Garlic also energizes the system, stimulates the brain, and dispels fatigue.

  1   **4½- to 5-pound fresh ham, shank or butt, preferably organic**
10   **cloves garlic, peeled**
      Sea salt
      Ground pepper
  2   **cups unsweetened applesauce (optional)**

1. Position the oven shelves to fit the ham in the center. Preheat the oven to 425 degrees.

2. Using a sharp paring knife, cut ten 1-inch crosscut openings all around the ham. In each opening, put a clove of garlic, salt, and pepper. Then sprinkle salt and pepper generously all over the exterior.

3. Place the ham in a deep baking pan and put it into the oven. Reduce the

(Garlic-roasted Fresh Ham—Continued)

heat to 350 degrees. Cook until no pink juices run when the ham is deeply pricked with a large fork, or until the internal temperature reaches 160 degrees on a meat thermometer.

4. Remove the ham from the oven. Allow it to rest for 5 to 10 minutes, covered with a sheet of parchment paper.

5. Carve the ham in thin slices and place on a hot serving platter. Serve immediately with applesauce on the side and any of your favorite fixings. *Kalé Órxie!* (Enjoy a good appetite!)

Cooking Tip: Slice leftover ham into thin pieces and use over a period of days for sandwiches, or cut leftovers into chunks and add to soup. If the roast has a bone, you can make a stock with it or add it when cooking beans to add a rich smoky flavor and PMS-alleviating nutrients such as calcium.

Nutritional Stars: Vitamin B6, vitamin B12, folic acid, iron

 # Braised Lamb Shanks with Garlic

Yield: 4 to 6 servings

Here's a simple way to tone down the strong flavors of lamb while adding a delicious garlicky Mediterranean taste.

PMS Benefits: Lamb provides selenium, a trace mineral that enhances the benefits of vitamin E. Premenstrual women with sufficient vitamin E experience less fatigue and fewer headaches.

  3 lamb shanks, preferably organic
  2 tablespoons extra-virgin olive oil
10 cloves garlic, unpeeled
  1 teaspoon dried rosemary
  2 teaspoons sea salt
¼ teaspoon ground pepper
  4 potatoes, peeled and cut in half
½ cup purified water
¼ cup cider vinegar

1. Wash the shanks under cold running water. Using paper toweling, dry them thoroughly.

2. Heat the olive oil in a large sauté pan on a medium flame. Brown the lamb shanks on all sides, uncovered, using tongs to turn them as they brown.

3. Add the garlic cloves with the rosemary, salt, and pepper. Cover and cook on low heat until almost tender, about 45 minutes. Turn the shanks over two or three times during the cooking.

4. Add the potatoes and ¼ cup water. Bring to a boil, covered. Reduce heat and cook until the potatoes are soft when pierced with a fork, about 15 minutes.

5. Turn the heat to high and allow the pan to get very hot. Mix the remaining ¼ cup water and the vinegar, and pour over the lamb and potatoes. Immediately cover to allow the vinegar to infuse the lamb.

6. Place the lamb shanks on a serving platter and carve some of the meat off the bone. Surround the lamb with the potatoes and garlic and drizzle the pan juices over the meat. Serve with a salad and a hearty appetite.

Cooking Tip: Neck bones, cubed meat, or other cuts of lamb can be substituted for lamb shanks. Chicken is also delicious cooked in this style.

Nutritional Stars: Vitamin B3, vitamin B12, vitamin C, vitamin E, folic acid, iron, selenium, zinc

 ## Midwestern Slow-cooking Lamb Pot Roast

Yield: 4 servings

Here's a no-fuss roast you can cook in a pot on top of the stove. The long cooking tenderizes the lamb, which fully absorbs the flavors of simple herbs.

PMS Benefits: Lamb contains vitamins B12 and B6. Vitamin B12 prevents a form of anemia and aids in the digestion and absorption of PMS-friendly foods. Vitamin B6 participates in the conversion of certain fats to prostaglandins, hormonelike compounds that can reduce menstrual cramping.

- 4 **tablespoons unsalted butter, preferably organic, or extra-virgin olive oil**
- ½ **cup whole-grain flour**
- ½ **teaspoon sea salt**
- ¼ **teaspoon ground pepper**
- 1 **2½- to 3-pound lamb shoulder roast, preferably organic**
- 2 **cups homemade salt-free stock**
- 2 **cloves garlic, chopped**
- 1 **bay leaf**

(Midwestern Slow-cooking Lamb Pot Roast—Continued)

1. Heat the butter or olive oil in a large Dutch oven.

2. In a large bowl or on a plate, mix the flour with the salt and pepper. Coat the lamb roast with the seasoned flour and place in the Dutch oven. Reserve the flour. Cook until golden brown. Using tongs or a large fork, turn the roast over and brown on the other side.

3. Sprinkle the remaining flour around the roast in the hot fat. Stir and cook for 30 seconds. Stir in the stock. Add the garlic and bay leaf, cover, and bring to a boil. Lower the flame and simmer until the meat is tender and beginning to fall apart, 1½ to 2½ hours, depending on the thickness and cut of meat. Add more stock, if needed.

4. Remove bay leaf. Place the roast on a serving platter and serve with a salad and mashed potatoes. Pour the pan juices into a gravy boat and drizzle on top of the potatoes.

Cooking Tip: If you've run out of stored stock in your freezer, it is easy to make some using a few vegetables and water. To 2 quarts purified water, add 1 onion, 2 carrots, 2 stalks celery, 3 peppercorns, and a bay leaf. Bring to a boil, reduce the flame, and simmer for 20 to 30 minutes. Strain and discard the vegetables—the stock is now ready for use.

Nutritional Stars: B-complex vitamins, vitamin B12, vitamin C, vitamin E, iron, zinc

Starting the Day

Hot and Cold Breakfast Cereals

Breakfast Grains and Quick Items

Eggs for Breakfast and Brunch

Breakfast Drinks

Reasons for Eating Breakfast

Breakfast is an important meal because it gives you the fuel you need to keep going all day. When you hit the premenstrual phase of your cycle, breakfast plays a more vital role in your routine because it contains many vitamins and minerals that ease the effects of PMS. Whole grains contain the B complex, fresh fruit has vitamin C, and special herbal teas can have a medicinal effect. For complex carbohydrates, enjoy some whole-grain toast, a homemade corn muffin, or pita bread with all-fruit conserves. Smear on some almond butter for protein and add a hot cup of herbal tea or a glass of freshly squeezed orange juice. Or try some whole-grain waffles or pancakes with freshly sliced fruit. Attack last night's leftovers and enjoy the added protein in a bowl of bean soup.

Avoid Headaches

If you skip breakfast or allow too much time to pass between meals, your blood sugar will drop and you'll be more prone to developing a bad headache. When the supply of glucose is lower than normal in the blood, the brain adapts by dilating blood vessels to increase blood flow. This allows more blood glucose to reach the brain cells, but it can also increase pressure and trigger pain. Even as little as a five percent drop in blood sugar can bring on a hypoglycemic headache. To avoid premenstrual hypoglycemia, eat at regular intervals throughout the day, and avoid foods such as sugars and refined grains that can cause your blood-sugar levels to fluctuate.

Sensitivities to certain foods can provoke headaches, especially migraines. Often the attack occurs twelve to thirty-six hours after the stomach has digested the food and substances called vasodilating amines dilate the blood vessels in the brain. Blood surges into the head and a person will feel a throbbing pain. During the premenstrual phase, five to ten days before menses, a woman who is inclined to migraines is even more sensitive to these amines. These compounds are particularly high in aged cheeses, alcohol, and chocolate. Other common food sensitivities can be triggered by citrus fruits, pork, meats, including sausage and hot dogs that contain sodium nitrate, and alcohol, especially champagne and red wine. The flavor enhancer MSG (monosodium glutamate), an ingredient common in Chinese foods, preserved and deli meats, and meat tenderizers, can also provoke headaches.

Simple and Speedy Morning Meals

Here are recommendations for easy and on-the-run breakfast foods that provide more nutrients than toast and coffee—or eating nothing at all!

- Whole-grain bread, almond or cashew butter, and all-fruit conserves—an updated PB&J sandwich.
- Bran, corn, or blueberry muffins made with whole-grain flours and no refined sugars.
- Eggs, in any style (soft or hard-boiled, scrambled, or sunny-side) and sesame whole wheat pita.
- Hot cereals such as oatmeal or any creamed cereal such as wheat, rye, kasha, or corn grits.
- Premeasured hot cereals without refined sugar.
- Plain yogurt with living cultures and sliced fresh fruit or all-fruit conserves.
- Cold cereal. All of your childhood favorites can now be found with low salt, no added sugar, intact fiber, and no preservatives at your local natural-food store.
- Leftover cornmeal, Polenta Cups (see page 92) browned in butter, sprinkled with cinnamon, and drizzled with pure maple syrup.

Filling Fruit Meals

Fruit for breakfast is a refreshing way to introduce vitamins, minerals, and enzymes into your system. The natural fluids in fruit also helps to dispel fatigue, a common symptom of PMS. Here are some nutrient-rich and easy combinations:

- Fresh cantaloupe, mango, and papaya chunks with blackberries.
- Fresh pear slices cooked in unsweetened apricot juice with currants and a cinnamon stick, and topped with roasted pecans.
- Dried apricots and peaches (unsulphured preferred), stewed in unsweetened apple juice with sunflower seeds or almonds.
- Add chopped, unsweetened, and unsulphured dried fruit to your hot or cold breakfast cereals. Try apricots, peaches, pineapple, prunes, apples, pears, raisins, currants, banana, papaya, and even mango.
- Add almonds, walnuts, or sunflower seeds for a heartier fruit minimeal.

Breakfast Protein: Eggs, Fish, and Meats

Eating protein at breakfast keeps you from feeling hungry by 10:00 A.M. While eating eggs is the most common way to add substance to the meal, they are usually not recommended for a PMS diet as they can trigger various symptoms in sensitive women. In this section, we do include recipes and health tips for cooking eggs, should you find that you can tolerate them, and to stimulate your cooking creativity when you are cooking for others.

Some women find that eating meat increases painful menstrual cramps, but if you can tolerate it, there are various kinds to choose from. You can purchase many breakfast meats without sugar and preservatives that worsen PMS symptoms. Look for bacon without the nitrites, chemical-free sausages, and cured meats made with lean chicken or turkey.

If eggs and meat are off your list, there is a quick and easy way to add protein to breakfast by including ready-to-eat fish such as canned salmon and herring, or fish from last night's dinner. The oils of these and other fish are high in essential fatty acids that ease menstrual cramping, and reduce fluid retention and irritability.

- Cooked salmon, white fish, herring, or cod with a garnish of capers, lemon juice, and flaxseed oil on crackers or in an omelet.
- Organic chicken livers cooked with a little butter and seasoned with sea salt and pepper, served on toast with caramelized onions.
- Savory patties made with ground turkey or pork, sage, garlic, and sea salt. Shape the patties and cook them in a skillet until golden on both sides. Add several patties to eggs, or just slide them into a warmed whole-grain pita bread. Make patties ahead and freeze.

Whole-Grain Hot and Cold Cereals

The natural-food store carries many whole-grain hot cereals that can be cooked in 5 or 10 minutes, such as creamy brown rice cereals and ground kasha. Grain flakes, such as barley, millet, rye, rice, and wheat, provide interesting tastes and variety. Oatmeal, the old standby, takes 20 minutes to cook (we do not recommend the quick-cooking variety). Granola (baked oat cereal) and muesli (raw oat cereal) can be eaten cooked or uncooked, or soaked overnight in plain yogurt. When you shop for cereal and granola, read the labels, and be on the lookout for brands loaded with sugars. The natural-food store will have the best selection of the healthiest items.

Take a close look at the cold cereals in the natural-food store. These days you can find cereals with no added or artificial sugars, preservatives, or chemical food colorings, substances that can potentially disturb your blood sugar and monthly cycle. Look for your childhood favorites now made with quality ingredients, such as oat circles, wheat and corn flakes, crispies made with brown rice, and whole-grain puffed cereals.

Cook hot cereals in water and add cinnamon, butter, and a pinch of sea salt. For cold cereals, rice, almond, or other grain and nut milks, or apple juice are the most common liquid additions if you need to cut cow's milk out of your diet. If you regularly consume milk, and dairy doesn't trigger menstrual symptoms such as cramps, use the organic varieties of milk, plain yogurt, buttermilk, or a little diluted cream.

Medicinal Herbal Teas for PMS

Try caffeine-free herbal teas, grain coffee substitutes, and hot spiced cider. Stopping a moment for a cup of tea has benefits well beyond quenching the thirst, especially if the tea is made with one of the many herbs traditionally used by women to ease menstrual pain, such as red raspberry leaf, licorice, and black cohosh.

Herbs that are tonics for the uterus include blue cohosh, chasteberry, rue, and false unicorn root, which normalize the menstrual cycle. Other herbs treat various types of premenstrual syndrome. Tea made from the common herb chamomile can ease anxiety. A more potent and calming brew is made with equal parts valerian and skullcap. Alleviate your depression with rosemary, lavender, lemon balm, damiana, and vervain. Dandelion, celery seeds, and juniper berries are effective diuretics that reduce fluid retention associated with PMS. Ginger relieves fatigue associated with PMS and also eases menstrual cramps by relaxing your muscles. Cramp bark also prevents muscle spasms.

Teas sold as menstrual tonics usually contain a variety of healing herbs. You can also buy dried herbs and create your own mixtures. While herbs do contain active ingredients that can affect body chemistry, herbal teas are mild therapies that normally contain low concentrations. Should you experience side effects, such as stomach upset and intestinal problems, immediately stop taking the herb. However, taking herbs normally presents no risks beyond certain individual sensitivities. These recommended herbs have withstood the test of time, as there is a long tradition of women tending to their needs through the use of medicinal plants.

Avoid caffeinated and decaffeinated beverages of any kind, and drinks made with refined sugars or chemical sweeteners.

Please see the Appendix for "Brands We Trust," page 238.

 # Hot Oatmeal with Cinnamon and Raisins

Yield: 4 servings   100% vegetarian

There's no better way to start off the day than with a bowl of hot oatmeal, which contains many of the nutrients you need to keep your PMS at bay.

PMS Benefits: Complex carbohydrates take a long time to break down into glucose, so they provide a steady flow of blood sugar over several hours and prevent symptoms such as increased appetite and headaches. Whole grains also add zinc, magnesium, and calcium, which steady moods and promote restful sleep. These great-for-you complex carbohydrates include whole-meal breads and flours, brown rice, and whole-grain breakfast cereals such as the oatmeal in this recipe.

> **2 cups purified water**
> **1 cup rolled oatmeal (see Note)**
> **¼ cup unsulphured raisins or currants**
> **1 teaspoon cinnamon or 1 cinnamon stick**
> **½ teaspoon sea salt**
> **2 to 3 tablespoons pure maple syrup or honey (optional)**
> **1 tablespoon unsalted butter, preferably organic**
> **½ cup plain yogurt with active cultures, preferably organic**
> **¼ cup raw hazelnuts, almonds, or walnuts, chopped (optional)**
> **Fruit such as sliced strawberries, apples, bananas, or pears; fresh blueberries, raspberries, or blackberries; or a spoonful of all-fruit conserves**

1. In a medium-sized saucepan, put the water, oatmeal, raisins or currants, cinnamon, and salt. Bring to a boil, uncovered. Stir, lower flame, and simmer 20 minutes with the lid partly uncovered.

2. Add the maple syrup or honey if using, and butter. Stir and cook another 1 or 2 minutes to allow the butter to melt. Stir again before serving. Remove cinnamon stick, if used.

3. Spoon into large individual bowls. Top with 2 tablespoons yogurt for each serving and sprinkle with 1 tablespoon hazelnuts, almonds, or walnuts, if using, and any of the fruit suggestions.

Cooking Tip: For creamy oatmeal, start with cold water as we have done in this recipe. For a more chewy texture, bring the water to a boil first, add the oatmeal, and then continue with the procedure.

Note: Many whole grains such as millet, rye, wheat, or barley are available in a rolled or flaked form. Ask in your health-food store for the ones they carry.

Nutritional Stars: Vitamin B5, vitamin E, choline, inositol, magnesium

Helene's Heirloom Granola

Yield: 6 cups   100% vegetarian

This recipe comes from Good Breads, a bakery Lissa and a college friend owned in Illinois. We've cut it down from 25 pounds of rolled oats to 4 cups!

PMS Benefits: Women with PMS should avoid refined cereal grains that can lower levels of sugar in the blood, triggering such symptoms as sweating, palpitations, anxiety attacks, headaches, and continued cravings for sweet foods. Eating a complex carbohydrate such as whole-meal flour products, brown rice, potatoes, rye cereals, and oatmeal every 3 to 4 hours during the day can help to avoid these symptoms. Carry some of this granola with you for a midday snack.

- **4 cups rolled oatmeal**
- **½ cup raw walnuts, chopped coarsely**
- **½ cup raw almonds, chopped coarsely**
- **½ cup sesame seeds (see Cooking Tip 2)**
- **2 teaspoons cinnamon**
- **¼ cup unsalted butter or ghee (see page 227), preferably organic**
- **¼ to ½ cup pure maple syrup or honey**
- **¼ cup unsulphured blackstrap molasses**
- **½ teaspoon sea salt**
- **1 cup purified water or unsweetened apple juice (see Note)**
- **½ cup unsweetened apple butter or applesauce**
- **1 teaspoon pure vanilla or almond extract**
- **Grated zest of 1 lemon or orange or 2 tablespoons bottled dried zest, preferably organic**
- **1 to 2 cups unsulphured dried fruit, such as raisins, currants, or dried blueberries, apricot bits, apple pieces, or chopped prunes**

1. Position the oven racks to fit several baking sheets with sides. Preheat the oven to 350 degrees.

2. In a large bowl, combine the oatmeal, walnuts, almonds, sesame seeds, and cinnamon.

3. In a medium-sized saucepan, melt the butter or ghee on medium heat. Turn off flame. Add the maple syrup or honey, molasses, and salt, and stir well. Add the water or juice, apple butter or applesauce, and vanilla or almond extract. Stir again.

4. Pour the butter mixture into the oatmeal and stir well.

5. Spread the oatmeal onto the baking sheets. Place the sheets in the oven and bake until golden brown and crispy, 15 to 20 minutes. Using a spoon or a spatula, stir the granola as it bakes to prevent burning (especially around the corners and edges), about every 5 minutes.

6. Remove the baking sheets from the oven and pour the granola into a large bowl. Add the zest and dried fruit, toss, and set aside to cool completely.

7. When completely cool, store the granola in a covered container. It stays freshest if it is kept in the refrigerator or freezer.

Cooking Tip 1: For easier cleanup, line the pans with parchment paper.

Cooking Tip 2: Substitute or add unsweetened coconut, pumpkinseeds, flaxseeds, or chopped raw pecans or hazelnuts.

Note: The granola will be sweeter when made with apple juice.

Nutritional Stars: Vitamin B5, vitamin B6, vitamin E, choline, inositol, calcium, iron, magnesium, omega-3 fatty acids

Whole-Grain Pancakes with Peach Sauce

Yield: 4 servings   100% vegetarian

Add a little more flour to this pancake batter and voilà—waffle batter!

PMS Benefits: Whole grains contain a full range of the B vitamins that are very important for your body when you are experiencing PMS symptoms, such as mood swings, irritability, and depression. (B vitamins help you to remain calm and resilient.) B-complex vitamins can be found in fruits, vegetables, beans, and whole grains.

The sauce:

2 cups unsweetened peach or apricot juice
¼ cup all-fruit conserves or pure maple syrup
   Pinch sea salt
¼ cup arrowroot or 3 tablespoons kuzu powder (see page 228)
¼ cup purified water
1 ripe peach or 3 apricots, pitted and chopped

(Whole-Grain Pancakes with Peach Sauce—Continued)

The pancakes:

2   **cups whole wheat pastry flour**
2   **teaspoons baking powder**
1   **teaspoon cinnamon**
½   **teaspoon sea salt**
1   **egg, preferably organic**
1   **to 1½ cups plain yogurt with active cultures, preferably organic**
½   **to ¾ cup purified water**
1   **cup fresh blueberries (optional)**
1   **or 2 peeled bananas, chopped (optional)**
2   **teaspoons grated orange zest (optional)**
    Unsalted butter, preferably organic (optional)

The sauce:

1. In a medium-sized saucepan, heat the juice, conserves or maple syrup, and salt. Bring to a boil, uncovered.

2. In a small bowl, mix the arrowroot or kuzu with ¼ cup water. Pour into the hot juice, and stir constantly until the juice thickens slightly and clears. Cook another 30 seconds.

3. Add the chopped fruit and cook another 1 or 2 minutes. The fruit topping is now ready to use. Keep covered to maintain warmth.

The pancakes:

1. Slowly preheat a pancake griddle or large cast-iron pan on low heat before mixing the batter.

2. In a large bowl, mix the flour, baking powder, cinnamon, and salt. In another bowl or blender, mix the egg, 1 cup yogurt, and ½ cup water. Pour the liquid ingredients into the dry and mix until just moistened. Stir in additional yogurt and water if needed to make a thick but pourable batter. (Add more yogurt and/or water to the mixture to thin, as needed. You should be able to pour the batter easily from a ladle or a measuring cup.)

3. Stir in any optional ingredients desired.

4. Turn the griddle heat to medium-high. Using very little butter, grease the griddle. If too much butter melts on the griddle, wipe excess off with a paper towel. Using a ladle or a measuring cup, pour pancake batter into 3-inch rounds, being careful to leave space between each. (As the batter pours, the pancake batter will spread until it begins cooking.) Cook until bubbles form on the top and begin to pop, about 1 minute. The bottoms will be golden. Using a metal spatula, carefully flip each pancake over and cook another minute.

5. Place the cooked pancakes on a platter and keep in a warm oven until all of the batter has been used.

6. Pour the peach sauce into a bowl with a small ladle. Serve the pancakes with the warm peach sauce on the side—and sit down to enjoy your labors.

Cooking Tip 1: For perfect pancakes, spread very little fat on the griddle before making each batch.

Cooking Tip 2: When cooking the pancake sauce, prevent the juices from getting too hot and suddenly boiling over by heating them in an uncovered saucepan.

Note: To make waffles, preheat the waffle grill according to the manufacturer's instructions. Using a ladle or measuring cup, pour pancake batter into medium-sized rounds, being careful to leave room between each. Cook until the bottoms are golden and bubbles have formed and are popping on the surface, about 1 minute. Using a metal spatula, flip them over and cook another minute. Serve hot.

Nutritional Stars: B-complex vitamins, vitamin E, calcium, iron, magnesium, zinc

 # Walnut-Ginger Quick Bread

Yield: 1 loaf   100% vegetarian

Here is a gingery bread made with mineral-rich blackstrap molasses. A fast and easy breakfast, travel snack, or a "sweet" at night, the muffins can be made ahead of time and refrigerated or kept frozen.

PMS Benefits: Blackstrap molasses contains calcium, iron, potassium, vitamin B6, vitamin E, magnesium, copper, inositol, para-aminobenzoic acid (PABA), and riboflavin. Calcium, magnesium, and potassium are vital to maintain healthy nerves and alleviate such symptoms as irritability and mood swings.

½ **cup unsalted butter, preferably organic, at room temperature**
½ **cup unsulphured blackstrap molasses**
½ **cup pure maple syrup**
 1 **cup plain yogurt with active cultures, preferably organic**
 1 **egg, preferably organic**
¼ **cup purified water**
½ **teaspoon sea salt**
2½ **cups whole wheat pastry flour**

(Walnut-Ginger Quick Bread—Continued)
    1 **cup raw walnuts, chopped coarsely**
    ½ **cup unsulphured raisins or currants (optional)**
    1 **to 2 tablespoons ground ginger**
    1 **teaspoon baking soda**
    1 **teaspoon cinnamon**

1. Position the oven racks to fit a loaf pan. Preheat the oven to 350 degrees.

2. Using a teaspoon or less of butter, grease a 9 × 5-inch loaf pan.

3. In a medium-sized bowl, using a whisk or in a food processor, beat the remaining butter until fluffy, 1 or 2 minutes. Add the molasses, maple syrup, yogurt, egg, water, and salt, and beat well.

4. In a large bowl, mix together the flour, ¾ cup walnuts, raisins or currants, ginger, soda, and cinnamon. Mix the liquid ingredients into the flour mixture and stir just until moistened. (If using a processor, add the walnuts and raisins after mixing the dry and liquid together.)

5. Pour the batter into the prepared loaf pan and top with the remaining ¼ cup walnuts. Bake the bread 50 to 60 minutes. When done, it will pull away slightly from the sides of the pan.

6. Take the quick bread out of the oven and allow to cool for 10 minutes in the pan. Slide a knife around the sides of the bread to loosen. Transfer the loaf to a wire rack to continue cooling.

7. When cool, using a serrated knife, slice the bread. Store the bread in a plastic bag in the refrigerator or freezer.

Cooking Tip: When making baked goods, dissolve salt by adding it to the wet ingredients.

Nutritional Stars: B-complex vitamins, vitamin E, calcium, copper, iron, potassium, magnesium, zinc

Oatmeal-Prune Muffins with Sunflower Tops

Yield: 12 muffins   100% vegetarian

These muffins are packed with whole grain, fruit, and seeds, and we guarantee they'll satisfy your sweet tooth.

PMS Benefits: An iron deficiency can cause anemia, a heavy monthly flow, and fatigue. When you need reviving, try prunes, which contain iron.

½ **cup unsulphured pitted prunes**
¼ **cup unsweetened apple juice**
½ **cup unsalted butter, preferably organic, at room temperature**
¾ **cup pure maple syrup or honey**
¼ **cup unsulphured blackstrap molasses**
1 **cup plain yogurt with active cultures, preferably organic**
1 **egg, preferably organic**
¼ **cup purified water**
½ **teaspoon sea salt**
2½ **cups whole wheat pastry flour**
1 **cup rolled oatmeal**
 Grated zest of 1 orange or 2 tablespoons bottled
  dry zest, preferably organic
1 **teaspoon cinnamon**
1 **teaspoon baking soda**
1 **teaspoon nutmeg**
½ **cup raw sunflower seeds**

1. Position the oven racks to fit a muffin pan. Preheat the oven to 350 degrees.

2. In a small saucepan, bring the prunes and apple juice to a boil, covered. Reduce heat and simmer until softened, about 5 minutes.

3. Using a teaspoon of butter or less, grease a muffin pan or line each cup with a paper muffin cup.

4. Place a sieve in a bowl and drain the prunes, saving the liquid. After the prunes have cooled, chop coarsely.

5. In a medium-sized bowl, using a whisk, or in a food processor, beat the remaining butter until fluffy, 1 or 2 minutes. Add the maple syrup or honey, molasses, yogurt, egg, water, and salt and beat well. Stir in the prunes and remaining prune liquid.

6. In a separate bowl, mix together the flour, oatmeal, orange zest, cinnamon, baking soda, and nutmeg. Stir well.

(Oatmeal-Prune Muffins with Sunflower Tops—Continued)

7. Mix the liquid and dry ingredients together, just until moistened.

8. Fill the prepared muffin cups three-fourths full. Top with the sunflower seeds. Bake the muffins until golden on top, 20 to 25 minutes.

9. Take the muffins out of the oven and place on a wire rack to cool—or if you can't wait, eat them right away! (With a cup of caffeine-free tea.)

10. Store the cooled muffins in a plastic bag. They will stay the freshest if stored in the refrigerator or freezer.

Cooking Tip: The pitted prunes can be replaced with ½ cup unsulphured raisins or if you prefer sweeter muffins, add them both.

Nutritional Stars: Vitamin A, B-complex vitamins, vitamin E, iron

Lemon–Poppy Seed Muffins or Loaf

Yield: 1 loaf or 12 muffins   100% vegetarian

Turn a muffin recipe into a loaf or a loaf into a tray of muffins. Here we give you both options for this delicious cake filled with lemon zest and poppy seeds.

PMS Benefits: Stock up on several kinds of seeds, such as sesame, pumpkin, or the poppy seeds featured in this recipe. As seeds are future plants, even small amounts deliver significant quantities of vitamins and minerals. A teaspoon of poppy seeds adds a good amount of calcium, which tends to decline during the two weeks before menstruation begins.

  ½ **cup unsalted butter, preferably organic, at room temperature**
  1 **cup pure maple syrup or honey**
  1 **cup plain yogurt with active cultures, preferably organic**
  1 **egg, preferably organic**
    Juice and grated zest of 2 lemons, preferably organic
  ½ **teaspoon sea salt**
1½ **cups whole wheat pastry flour**
  1 **cup high-lysine cornmeal or additional whole wheat pastry flour**
  ¼ **cup poppy seeds**
  1 **teaspoon baking soda**
  ½ **teaspoon cinnamon**

1. Position the oven racks to fit a muffin or loaf pan. Preheat the oven to 350 degrees. Grease or line the pan of your choice with parchment paper or paper-cup liners.

2. Using a teaspoon of butter or less, grease a 9 × 5-inch loaf pan, or place paper baking cups in a muffin pan.

3. In a medium-sized bowl with a whisk, or in a food processor, beat the remaining butter until fluffy, 1 or 2 minutes. Add the maple syrup or honey, yogurt, egg, lemon juice and zest, and salt, and beat well.

4. In a separate bowl, mix together the flour, cornmeal, poppy seeds, baking soda, and cinnamon. (If using the processor, add the poppy seeds after combining the dry and liquid ingredients.) Mix the liquid and dry ingredients together, stirring just enough to moisten.

5. Pour the batter into the prepared loaf pan or fill the muffin cups three-fourths full. Bake the bread 50 to 60 minutes, or the muffins 20 to 25 minutes. When done, the bread or muffins will pull away slightly from the sides of the pan and be golden on top.

6. Take the quick bread or muffins out of the oven. Allow the bread to cool for 10 minutes or—eat the muffins right away!

7. When cool, using a serrated knife, slice the loaf. Store in a plastic bag in the refrigerator or freezer.

Cooking Tip: When making a quick bread or muffins, mix the liquid and dry ingredients together just enough to moisten. This keeps the batter from over-developing and yielding a tough baked product.

Nutritional Stars: Vitamin A, vitamin E, calcium, magnesium, zinc

 # Flip-less Sunny-side Over

Yield: 1 serving   100% vegetarian

This technique uses the least amount of fat while cooking the yolk ever so gently— plus it saves you from a broken yolk!

PMS Benefits: While some women with PMS find that eggs worsen menstrual cramps, eggs are a good source of balanced protein. Eggs also contain zinc and vitamin A, which work together to heal acne, a monthly problem for many teenagers and some adults.

1 **teaspoon unsalted butter, preferably organic**
2 **eggs, preferably organic**
1 **tablespoon purified water**

(Flip-less Sunny-side Over—Continued)

   1. On a medium flame, heat a skillet and melt the butter. Swish the butter around to coat the entire bottom.

   2. Crack open each egg and carefully allow it to slide out of the shell and into the pan without breaking the yolk. Continue to cook until the white starts to set, about 30 seconds.

   3. Add the water to the pan and immediately cover. Keep covered (don't peek!) about 1 minute. This allows the water to form steam to further cook the whites of the eggs and create a slight film over the yolks.

   4. Using a spatula, cut and separate the eggs. Then gently slide the spatula under each egg to loosen it from the bottom of the skillet and remove it to a plate.

   5. Serve hot whole-grain toast, homemade muffins, or pita bread wedges alongside the eggs and enjoy your meal.

   Cooking Tip: Organic eggs usually have a dark orange yolk and a harder shell than commercial eggs, and when fresh will have a firm white that stays close to the yolk.

   Nutritional Stars: Vitamin A, vitamin E, folic acid, iron, zinc, omega-3 fatty acids

---

Soft-Boiled and Poached Eggs

   If you are not troubled by menstrual cramps, having eggs for breakfast from time to time is just fine. You may be concerned about the cholesterol in eggs, but there is some good news. Gently cooking eggs by soft boiling and poaching helps prevent the cholesterol in the yolks from damaging your arteries. Scrambling an egg oxidizes its cholesterol since it is exposed directly to high heat. Evidence shows that this oxidized cholesterol, not cholesterol itself, is the culprit in heart disease.

Frittata and Omelet Primer

Yield: 4 servings   100% vegetarian

Omelets and frittatas are fast and easy to make. They offer a hearty protein base for both savory and spicy fillings. Serve them with toasted whole-grain breads, such as multigrain slices, English muffins, sourdough bread, sesame pita, or homemade savory or sweet muffins, and a side of potatoes. Add a spicy turkey patty or sausage, along with a cup of herbal tea, for a real country breakfast.

PMS Benefits: Here's a chance to add variety to your meals by including novel ingredients to your omelets and frittatas, a range of foods which gives you an ample helping of nutrients for general menstrual help.

- **8 eggs, preferably organic (see Note)**
- **2 tablespoons purified water**
- **½ teaspoon herbal sea salt**
- **1 to 2 tablespoons unsalted butter, preferably organic**
   Any filling or topping desired (see page 180)

To make a frittata:

1. In a bowl or blender, lightly beat the eggs, water, and herbal sea salt.

2. Melt the butter in a 10- or 12-inch omelet pan (a skillet with sloping sides) over medium heat. Tilt the skillet in all directions to cover the entire bottom and about one-third of the way up the sides with butter.

3. Increase the heat and pour in the eggs. Begin cooking the eggs without stirring until they start to bubble around the edges, about 10 seconds. Into the center, carefully mix in the filling, being careful not to pierce the bottom where the eggs have cooked so as to keep the frittata in one piece. It should take about 3 minutes for the bottom to set.

4. Preheat the broiler and place the skillet under the heat until the frittata puffs up, becomes golden, and the eggs have fully set.

5. Slide a sharp knife around the edge of the pan, loosening the frittata from the sides. Carefully slide it out of the skillet and onto a plate.

To make an omelet:

1. In a bowl or blender, lightly beat 2 eggs, 1½ teaspoons water, and a pinch of herbal sea salt.

2. For individual omelets, melt 1 teaspoon butter in a 6- or 8-inch omelet pan (a skillet with sloping sides) over medium heat. Tilt the skillet in all directions to cover the entire bottom and about one-third of the way up the sides with butter.

(Frittata and Omelet Primer—Continued)

3. Increase the heat and pour in the eggs. Cook the eggs without stirring until they begin to bubble around the edges, about 10 seconds. Stir the center, being careful not to pierce the bottom where the eggs have cooked so as to keep the omelet in one piece. It should take about 1 minute for the bottom to set.

4. In a small skillet, warm the filling. Put the warm filling on half of the omelet. Carefully slide the omelet halfway onto the plate, then flip the other half over the bottom portion to form a half circle.

5. Place the plate in a warm oven and repeat for the three other omelets (or use four omelet pans at once).

Cooking Tip: For a very silky egg texture, pour the beaten eggs into the skillet through a sieve. Discard the white membranes and stringy parts.

Note: Omelets are beaten eggs that are cooked in a wide skillet and after setting are folded over with a filling inside the fold. Frittatas start out the same way but are left open in the shape of a large flat disk. The vegetables and meats are incorporated as the eggs are cooking or placed on top of the disk and then served from the pan.

Nutritional Stars: Vitamin A, choline, inositol, vitamin E, folic acid, iron, zinc, omega-3 fatty acids

Fillings and Toppings for Omelets and Frittatas

- Caviar, minced onion, and a touch of plain yogurt
- Caramelized onions and garlic, with golden potatoes
- Avocado slices, cherry tomatoes, and scallions
- Chives, reconstituted and chopped sun-dried tomatoes, fresh ricotta, and garlic
- Sautéed red and green bell peppers, and garlic
- Chèvre with minced parsley, dill, and fresh cilantro (coriander)
- Sautéed leeks, currants, and walnuts
- Pimento slices, garlic, and grated fresh mozzarella
- Sautéed portobello, porcini, and oyster mushrooms
- Red onion, with salmon and fresh basil
- Shallots, black olives, and anchovies
- Scallions, roasted or sautéed garlic, and grated fresh mozzarella or cheddar

And recipes from the book for fillings or top your eggs (a great way to use leftovers):

- Four-Onion and Red-Bean Vegetable Tagine (see page 41)
- Broccoli Salad with Red Onion and Black Olives (see page 54)
- Chickpea and Red Onion Hummus (see page 63)
- Texan Two-step Chili (see page 72)

- Caribbean Twice-cooked Pinto Beans with Plantains (see page 76)
- Spinach and Sweet Potato Sauté (see page 111)
- Ukrainian Cabbage and Potatoes with Fresh Herbs (see page 120)
- Fast Salmon with Lemon, Garlic, and Capers (see page 134)
- Garlic-roasted Fresh Ham (see page 159)

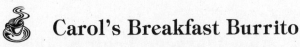

Carol's Breakfast Burrito

Yield: 4 servings   100% vegetarian

It can't get simpler than this! Corn or whole wheat tortillas wrapped around scrambled eggs, and whatever else you'd like. On ski trips, we downed these each morning before rushing to the slopes—a real hit with the ski-house crew.

PMS Benefits: The fiber in the whole-grain tortillas clears out excess estrogen, reducing tenderness and swelling in the breasts, as well as nervous tension.

8 eggs, preferably organic
2 tablespoons purified water
2 pinches sea salt
1 pinch ground pepper
1 tablespoon unsalted butter, preferably organic
4 corn or whole wheat tortillas
   Tasty additions (optional; see Note)

1. Break the eggs into a medium-sized bowl. Using a fork or whisk, beat the eggs until well mixed. Add the water, salt, and pepper, and mix again.

2. In a medium-sized skillet, on a moderate flame, melt the butter. Pour in the egg mixture and cook on a medium-low flame. Using a fork or spoon, stir the eggs as they cook. Add any other ingredients as desired (see Note).

3. Warm the tortillas directly on a flame in a heated cast-iron skillet, or in a toaster oven. Place one tortilla on each plate. (If you plan to season the tortillas, do so after they are heated.)

4. Evenly divide the cooked eggs and place them on top of the tortillas. Let each person roll his or her tortilla up and eat away! Serve with a cup of hot peppermint tea—and you're ready to head out for the day!

Cooking Tip: After heating the tortillas, we sometimes like to butter them lightly and sprinkle with salt and pepper.

(Carol's Breakfast Burrito—Continued)

Note: Tasty additions can include any favorite leftover bean, chicken, or fish recipe, grated raw milk cheese (organic preferred), salsa, twice-cooked beans, caramelized onions, or a few squirts of hot sauce.

Nutritional Stars: Vitamin A, B-complex vitamins, vitamin E, calcium, iron, magnesium, zinc, omega-3 fatty acids

 # Flaxseed Fruit Shake

Yield: 2 shakes   100% vegetarian

Similar to lassi, an Indian drink that blends yogurt with fruit, our fruit shake has the added appeal of a very good source of fiber and essential omega-3 fatty acids.

PMS Benefits: Flaxseeds are very high in omega-3 fatty acids from which the body produces compounds that ease menstrual cramping and discomfort.

    4   to 6 tablespoons raw flaxseeds (see Note)
    2   cups unsweetened apple or apricot juice
    ½   cup plain yogurt with living cultures, preferably organic
    4   to 6 fresh or frozen strawberries, green stems removed

1. In a dry blender, grind the flaxseeds to a powder. (This can also be done in a clean spice grinder.)

2. Add the apple or apricot juice, yogurt, and strawberries. Blend until very smooth. Pour into tall glasses and add a straw.

Cooking Tip: When using frozen fruit choose the kinds that have no added sugar. Organic sugar-free fruits are also available.

Note: Start with 4 tablespoons and if the texture is enjoyable, the next time you make the shake use 6 tablespoons of flaxseeds.

Nutritional Stars: Vitamin B1, vitamin B6, vitamin B12, calcium, magnesium, omega-3 fatty acids

Banana and Fresh Fruit Smoothie

Yield: 2 smoothies   100% vegetarian

This nutritious, easy-to-digest smoothie will soothe your hunger.

PMS Benefits: Bananas contain vitamin B6, which is important for regulating many PMS symptoms, including fluid retention, breast tenderness, irritability, mood swings, bloating, and fatigue. Note that women who use birth-control pills may have lower vitamin B6 levels, so be sure to try other good sources of this vitamin such as chicken, turkey, beans, whole grains, salmon, tuna, nuts, and organic beef liver.

   2 **ripe bananas, cut into quarters**
   4 **fresh or frozen strawberries, green stems removed**
1½ **cups unsweetened apple juice**
   1 **ripe peach, pitted, or ½ cup fresh-cut pineapple**
   4 **ice cubes**
   2 **tablespoons raw almond butter**

1. In a blender put the bananas, strawberries, apple juice, peach or pineapple, ice, and almond butter. Blend until smooth.

2. Pour into two tall glasses and add straws. Sip it down for a refreshing and light morning meal.

Cooking Tip: Bananas are ripe when the skins are completely yellow and covered with small brown spots.

Nutritional Stars: Vitamin B2, vitamin B3, vitamin B6, vitamin E, iron, calcium, magnesium, potassium

A Crust Above

Sandwiches

The Brown Bag

You know all the reasons why it was impossible to eat lunch—can't get out of the office, schedule too busy, it's raining out. . . . But preparing portable food for lunch or snacks can be fast and easy, and a handy way to use up leftovers. To travel with the food, look for a collapsible, lightweight insulated bag with a handle and enough room to hold lunch, a beverage, and a few snacks. A thermos with a wide mouth keeps soups and stews steaming hot. If you place some sprouts or lettuce leaves on both slices of bread before adding the filling, a sandwich will last for most of the day without becoming soggy from a slice of tomato or sauerkraut. Store your sandwich and other goodies in the office refrigerator until you eat, or keep your sandwich fresh with a small ice pack. It takes only a few minutes each day to plan and prepare your brown-bag food. You'll be able to feed yourself nutritious meals at work that help balance hormones and prevent PMS.

Fast and Easy Lunch and Snack Ideas

- Whole-grain English muffin and Chickpea and Red Onion Hummus (see page 63) or any bean spread on whole-grain bread.
- Whole-grain toast, a smear of mustard, and tomato slices. Wrap in plastic and tuck in your purse—there's nothing to spoil.
- Open-faced sandwiches with avocado, salad greens, and a slice of tomato with mustard—it's easy to find these sandwiches in a local shop.
- Sardines, red onion rings, and cucumber slices on hearty whole wheat bread.
- A thermos-full of satisfying bean soup with a hunk of whole-grain bread.
- A bean salad, a few wedges of pita bread, and a bottle of purified water.
- Egg sandwich on a toasted English muffin.
- Raw nuts and seeds, homemade muffin, cherry tomatoes, cucumber, and a bean dip.

And recipes from the book (a great way to use leftovers):

- Any bean and vegetable soup, such as Chunky Vegetable Minestrone with Cannellini Beans (see page 26).
- Last night's Cajun Red Lentil and Corn Stew (see page 37).
- Texan Two-step Chili (see page 72) with corn chips.
- A South African Navy Bean Croquette Logs (see page 78) sandwich in a whole wheat hot dog bun.
- Any of our *One Dozen Leafy Greens* (see page 103) such as Pickled Collards with Capers, Currants, and Walnuts (see page 116), in whole wheat pita bread.
- Leftover Fast Salmon with Lemon, Garlic, and Capers (see page 134) with a green salad.
- Walnut Oat Bars (see page 211).

Whole-Grain Sandwich-Bread Pointers

Choose quality whole-grain breads for your sandwiches. You can find a wide variety of breads without ever having to make a single loaf! Sliced whole-grain breads are available in whole wheat, multigrain, European-style (hearty and chewy), oatmeal, and also unsliced whole-grain sourdough and baguettes. You can also make sandwiches using whole-grain rolls, pita breads, English muffins, or croissants. Explore the variety of breads available to start your sandwich-making.

 # Spicy Cajun Grilled Chicken Sandwiches

Yield: 4 sandwiches

A fully flavored sandwich that will please almost any palate—and a great portable food for an office lunch or a picnic.

PMS Benefits: Chicken contains zinc, which helps to ease menstrual cramping, and a range of the B vitamins that can soothe menstrual nerves. Niacin plays a special role in keeping the skin healthy, as it promotes circulation, counteracting the acne that can develop as a woman begins her monthly cycle.

> 2 tablespoons extra-virgin olive oil, ghee (see page 227),
>   or unsalted butter, preferably organic
> 1 onion, sliced
> 2 cloves garlic, minced
> 4 boneless chicken breasts, preferably organic
> 2 teaspoons chili powder
> ½ teaspoon powdered mustard
> ½ teaspoon herbal sea salt
> ¼ teaspoon ground pepper and/or a dash of cayenne pepper
> 1 teaspoon fresh lemon juice
> 8 slices whole-grain bread or 4 whole-grain rolls
> 4 teaspoons prepared mustard
> 4 leaves Bibb or mizuna lettuce, washed
> 1 ripe tomato, sliced
> 4 kosher dill pickles

1. In a medium-sized skillet, heat the oil, ghee, or butter on high heat and add the onion. Lower the flame and cook uncovered until the onions begin to turn translucent, 2 or 3 minutes. Stir occasionally.

2. Add the garlic and chicken breasts. Sprinkle the chicken with the chili powder, mustard, herbal sea salt, and pepper and/or cayenne. Cover and continue cooking for another 5 minutes.

3. Turn the chicken breasts over and stir the onions. If the chicken is sticking to the bottom of the skillet, add several tablespoons of water. Cover and cook until the breasts are fully cooked, another 4 to 6 minutes.

4. Sprinkle with lemon juice, heat for 1 more minute, covered, and turn off flame.

5. To build the sandwiches: On a work surface, lay out four slices of whole-grain bread or the bottom halves of the rolls. Spread each with a teaspoon of mustard. Place a lettuce leaf on each slice of bread. (If the leaf is too big, tear or fold it to the proper size, still using the whole leaf.)

6. If you prefer, slice the cutlets into strips before placing them on top of the lettuce. Top the chicken with the cooked onion slices and a tomato slice. Cover each sandwich with the second slice of bread or the roll top, and serve with a pickle on the side. Great hot or cold.

Cooking Tip: Bottled Cajun spice mixes can be purchased to replace the chili powder, mustard, and pepper or cayenne.

Nutritional Stars: Vitamin A, B-complex vitamins, vitamin E, calcium, magnesium, iron, zinc, omega-3 fatty acids

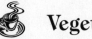 **Vegetarian Heros**

Yield: 4 heros   100% vegetarian

This hero is an easy way to get in several servings of vegetables in one meal.

PMS Benefits: Mushrooms contain high levels of pantothenic acid (vitamin B5), which is considered the "antistress vitamin." It plays a role in combating PMS-related fatigue by converting proteins, fats, and carbohydrates into energy. A deficiency in vitamin B5 can cause headache, nausea, and a tingling in the hands. Other foods that contain appreciable levels of pantothenic acid include beans, eggs, whole grains, avocado, bluefish and trout, and sunflower seeds.

1 **large portobello mushroom, stem removed**
3 **tablespoons extra-virgin olive oil or ghee (see page 227)**
2 **cloves garlic, sliced**
  Sea salt

(Vegetarian Heros—Continued)
    Purified water
½ **eggplant, cut into ¼- to ½-inch slices**
½ **teaspoon dried thyme, marjoram, basil, or oregano**
1 **zucchini, cut diagonally into ¼-inch slices**
1 **red onion, cut into ¼-inch rounds**
4 **whole-grain rolls or 2 whole-grain baguettes**
4 **teaspoons mustard**
1 **bunch watercress or arugula, ends trimmed, washed**
½ **cucumber, peeled and sliced thin**
½ **recipe The Best Onion-Garlic Dip-o-nnaise (see page 64)**
¼ **to ½ cup fresh sauerkraut**
4 **leaves lettuce, such as romaine or chicory, washed**

1. Under running water, quickly rinse the top of the mushroom, being careful not to get the underside of the mushroom wet. Use paper toweling to dry the top and set it aside. Trim the stem, wash, and cut it into four slices.

2. Heat a large skillet on a high flame and add 1 tablespoon oil or ghee. Place the mushroom cap in the skillet topside down and scatter the stem slices around it. Add the garlic and sprinkle with a pinch or two of salt. Lower the flame to medium, cover, and cook until the cap starts to release its juices, 3 to 4 minutes.

3. Turn the cap and stem slices over. Add 2 tablespoons water, cover, and continue cooking for another 4 minutes. Remove to a plate and set aside. When cool, slice the mushroom cap into eight to twelve slices.

4. To the same pan, on medium heat, add 2 more tablespoons water, 1 tablespoon oil or ghee, and the eggplant slices. Sprinkle with the herb of choice and several pinches of salt. (Or they can be broiled; see Cooking Tip below.) Cook covered for 2 minutes. Using a spatula, carefully turn each slice over. Add additional water, if needed. Cover and continue cooking for another 3 to 4 minutes. Carefully remove to a plate (the eggplant will be very soft) and set aside. Using the remaining oil, repeat this procedure with the zucchini and then the red onion, until all the vegetables have been cooked. The vegetables are now ready for sandwich fixings.

5. To build the sandwiches: On a work surface, cut open the rolls or baguettes and lay out the bottoms. Spread the bread bottoms with mustard and cover with three or four stems of watercress or arugula. Layer two or three slices mushroom, one to one and a half slices of eggplant, several slices of zucchini, and a mound of onion rings. Add the cucumber slices and a big dollup of The Best Onion-Garlic Dip-o-nnaise. Gather up the sauerkraut in your hand and squeeze out the liquid. Put some on each sandwich and top with a lettuce leaf. Cover the sandwiches with their top pieces. (If using baguettes, cut in half.) Insert a long toothpick to hold everything in place. Enjoy the gushing flavors!

Cooking Tip: Broiling these marinated vegetables will be just as tasty. Place the broiler shelf 3 to 4 inches away from the heat source, and broil the vegetables in a nonglass pan or on a cookie sheet.

Nutritional Stars: B-complex vitamins, vitamin B5, vitamin E, magnesium, zinc

 # Fresh Tuna Salad Sandwiches

Yield: 4 sandwiches

We've made this salad without commercially bottled mayonnaise, a source of poor-quality fats and unnecessary calories. You can also convert this recipe into egg, chicken, or shrimp salad.

PMS Benefits: Tuna contains vitamin B6, which helps to regulate a myriad of PMS symptoms, including mood swings, irritability, fluid retention, breast tenderness, bloating, sugar craving, and fatigue. Vitamin B6 is also found in whole grains, especially brown rice, beans, spinach and broccoli, mangoes, walnuts, sunflower seeds and flaxseeds, and trout.

The tuna salad:

- 3 or 4 tuna or salmon steaks or 1 fillet, ¾ to 1 pound (see Note)
- 2 tablespoons unsalted butter, preferably organic
- 4 tablespoons purified water
- 2 cloves garlic or 1 shallot, minced fine
- ½ teaspoon herbal sea salt
  Freshly ground white pepper
- 4 radishes or 2 scallions, ends trimmed, washed and minced
- 2 stalks celery, minced

The dressing:

- ¼ cup plain yogurt with active cultures, preferably organic
- 1 tablespoon extra-virgin olive oil
- 1 tablespoon flaxseed oil
- 2 teaspoons prepared mustard
- 2 tablespoons cider vinegar or lemon juice

(Fresh Tuna Salad Sandwiches—Continued)

The sandwiches:

8 slices whole-grain bread or 4 whole-grain rolls
4 leaves of radicchio or chicory, washed
4 pimento halves or pieces

The tuna salad:

1. Under cold running water, wash the fish steaks or fillets. Dry on paper toweling.

2. Heat 1 tablespoon butter and 2 tablespoons water in a large skillet. Place the fish in the pan and season with garlic, herbal sea salt, and several grinds of pepper. Cook 3 or 4 minutes. (For a grilled flavor, cook under the broiler.)

3. Using a spatula, turn the steaks over, add the remaining 1 tablespoon butter and 2 tablespoons water, and continue to sauté until the fish is thoroughly cooked and there is no pink left in the center.

4. Remove the fish to a plate to cool.

5. Using a knife and fork, cut the fish into thin slices and then cross-cut, making small pieces. (Or, if you prefer, with a fork flake the fish into small segments.) Remove and discard any bones.

6. Place the cut or flaked fish in a medium-sized bowl. Add the radishes or scallions and celery. Set aside to cool.

The dressing:

1. In a small bowl, stir together the yogurt, oils, mustard, and vinegar or lemon juice.

2. Pour the dressing over the flaked fish and stir well. Taste and season with additional salt and pepper, if needed.

The sandwiches:

On a work surface, lay out four slices of bread or the bottoms of the rolls. Put a leaf of radicchio or chicory on each. Place a scoop of tuna salad and a pimento half, or several pieces, on top. Cover the sandwiches with the remaining bread slices or roll tops. The sandwich is ready for munching or brown-bagging!

Cooking Tip: A short cut to making this fresh fish salad is to add one of our delicious dressings or favorite dips (dilute first), instead of the dressing suggestion we give for this recipe.

Note: To substitute for the tuna: Egg Salad—use 5 hard-cooked eggs that have been peeled and chopped; Chicken Salad—use 3 cups of shredded chicken (skinless white and/or dark meat). Proceed with Step 6.

Nutritional Stars: Vitamin B3, vitamin B6, vitamin E, calcium, magnesium, zinc, omega-3 fatty acids

Soft-shell Crab Sandwiches

Yield: 4 sandwiches

Crabs shed their hard outer shells from May through September, leaving the crab with a soft shell for about 6 hours. Due to their highly perishable nature, fresh soft-shell crabs are a specialty item in restaurants and fish markets. They are also an unusual food because they are eaten whole! Feast on the entire crab—legs, soft shell, and all, for a great source of calcium.

PMS Benefits: A deficiency in calcium can cause dysmenorrhea—cramps, nausea, vomiting, and lower back pain. High-calcium foods include dark, leafy greens such as bok choy and turnip greens, whole grains, blackstrap molasses, hazelnuts, figs, and yogurt.

4 **medium soft-shell crabs (see Note)**
½ **cup high-lysine corn flour or meal, or whole wheat flour**
½ **teaspoon sea salt**
¼ **teaspoon ground pepper**
4 **tablespoons unsalted butter, preferably organic**
2 **tablespoons extra-virgin olive oil or additional unsalted butter**
4 **cloves garlic, sliced**
¼ **bunch fresh parsley, leaves only, washed and minced**
1 **lemon, cut in half**
8 **slices whole-grain bread or 4 whole-grain rolls**
4 **teaspoons prepared mustard**
4 **lettuce leaves, such as romaine, Bibb, chicory, or other**
   favorite, washed

1. Fill a medium-sized bowl with cold water and add the crabs. Place in a colander in the sink. Remove the crabs one at a time, rinse under cold running water, and put in the colander to drain.

2. In a medium-sized bowl, stir the flour, salt, and pepper together. Dust each crab in the flour and set aside on a large plate, until all the crabs have been dusted.

3. In a skillet large enough to fit all the crabs at once, melt 2 tablespoons butter and 1 tablespoon olive oil on high heat. Add the crabs and garlic, and sprinkle all over with salt. Lower flame to medium, and cover the skillet with a splatter guard. Cook until the undersides of the crabs begin to turn pink, 3 to 4 minutes.

(Soft-shell Crab Sandwiches—Continued)

4. Using tongs, carefully turn the crabs over. Add the remaining butter and olive oil, and sprinkle with parsley. Continue cooking, covered by the splatter guard, until a fork can be inserted with little or no resistance, another 3 or 4 minutes.

5. Line a work surface with brown paper or toweling and place the cooked crabs on top to drain the excess fat. Squeeze half of the lemon over the crabs.

6. To build the sandwiches: On a work surface, lay out four slices of bread or the bottoms of the rolls. Spread 1 teaspoon of mustard on the bread. Put a leaf of romaine or Bibb lettuce on each and top with a hot or room-temperature soft-shell crab. (Be sure to serve some cooked parsley with each crab.) Cover the sandwiches with the remaining bread slices or roll tops. Cut the remaining lemon half into four pieces and serve a wedge on the side of each sandwich. Eat right away!

Cooking Tip: Use a splatter shield when cooking these crabs—or for anything else that splatters as it cooks to protect you from getting an oil burn.

Note: We prefer to purchase fresh crabs from a fishmonger as a last errand on a shopping trip. Have the crabs cleaned while you wait (eyes and gills are removed), and immediately take them home and refrigerate them. If possible, cook the crabs within hours of purchasing, or at least on the same day, because they spoil quickly. If the crabs are small, two per sandwich may be preferable.

Nutritional Stars: Vitamin B12, calcium, copper, magnesium, zinc

 # Open-faced French Lentil and Walnut Pâté Sandwiches

Yield: 4 sandwiches   100% vegetarian

Here's a ladies' lunch dish packed full of nutritious brain food—nuts, beans, and fresh herbs. Serve it with a knife and fork, some salad on the side, a cup of iced herbal tea, and a generous helping of good conversation.

PMS Benefits: Lentils contain folic acid, an effective relief for PMS depression, anxiety, and fatigue. Insufficient consumption of fresh vegetables and fruits or microwave cooking of these foods can cause a deficiency of folic acid. Folic acid works best when taken together with vitamin B12 and vitamin C.

2 cups French Dupuy or green lentils, sorted and washed (see page 71)
5 cups purified water
2 cloves garlic, peeled
1 onion, quartered
1 carrot, quartered
1 bay leaf
1 teaspoon dried marjoram
½ bunch fresh parsley, thick stems removed, washed, and chopped coarsely
1 tablespoon plus 4 teaspoons prepared mustard
2 teaspoons sea salt
½ teaspoon ground white pepper
¼ cup extra-virgin olive oil
½ to ¾ cup whole-grain bread crumbs
1 cup raw walnuts
4 slices hearty whole-grain bread or 4 whole-grain pita breads
4 lettuce leaves, such as romaine, Bibb, chicory, or other favorite, washed
4 tablespoons Yogurt Herb Dressing (see page 62, optional)
1 ripe tomato, sliced, or 8 reconstituted sun-dried tomatoes

1. In a large stockpot, put the lentils, water, garlic, onion, carrot, bay leaf, and marjoram. Bring to a boil, with the lid slightly uncovered. Reduce flame, cover the pot completely, and simmer until the lentils are soft, about 45 minutes. Stir occasionally.

2. Add the parsley, mustard, salt, and pepper and cook another 5 minutes. Remove the bay leaf and discard.

3. In a blender or food processor, add the cooked lentils, olive oil, bread crumbs, and walnuts. Pulse-chop just enough to chop the walnuts coarsely and blend. Do not overmix or puree.

4. Lightly oil a 9×5×3-inch loaf pan. Using a rubber spatula, spoon the pâté into the pan and smooth the top. Cover with plastic film and refrigerate for 3 to 4 hours or overnight.

5. Slide a knife blade around the edge of the loaf to loosen. Place a cutting board or large plate on top of the loaf pan and invert. Holding the loaf pan together with the board or plate, shake to release the pâté from the pan.

6. With a chef's knife, cut the loaf into ¾-inch slices. Wet the blade before cutting *each* slice. The pâté will mash slightly on cutting.

7. To build the sandwiches: In a toaster, lightly toast the bread slices or pitas just enough to warm them. On a work surface, lay out the bread and spread 1 teaspoon of mustard on each. Put a lettuce leaf on each. Top with a slice of pâté, a dollop of Yogurt Herb Dressing, and put one or two tomato slices or two sun-dried tomato halves on top—and voilà! Serve with a knife and fork.

(Open-faced French Lentil and Walnut Pâté Sandwiches—Continued)

Cooking Tip: French Dupuy lentils are small, round green beans that have a very delicate taste. They can be purchased in specialty stores or ordered by mail. When these beans are not available, green or red lentils will work fine.

Nutritional Stars: Vitamin B3, vitamin B5, vitamin B12, vitamin C, folic acid, magnesium, zinc

 ## Roasted and Marinated Tricolored Pepper Sandwiches with Chèvre

Yield: 4 sandwiches   100% vegetarian

We've created a sandwich that is chock-full of tasty pimento slices, dripping with the flavors of garlic, extra-virgin olive oil, and vinegar.

PMS Benefits: Red and yellow vegetables are high in vitamin A, which counteracts premenstrual acne and oily skin. Vitamin A can also be found in sweet potatoes, carrots, winter squash such as butternut and Hubbard, cantaloupes, and mangoes.

1 red bell pepper
1 yellow or orange bell pepper
1 green or purple bell pepper
2 cloves garlic, minced
¼ teaspoon dried mint, thyme, or basil
3 tablespoons extra-virgin olive oil or flaxseed oil
3 tablespoons cider vinegar
¼ teaspoon sea salt plus additional as needed
4 whole-grain pita breads or whole-grain English muffins
1 log chèvre or sheep's milk cheese, such as ricotta salata, about 4 ounces
   Handful mizuna or mesclun leaves, washed and dried
   Ground pepper (optional)
4 kosher dill pickles

1. To roast the peppers: Position the broiler rack about 3 inches from the heat source. Preheat the broiler.

2. Place the peppers on a nonglass baking tray under the broiler. Roast until the tops have blackened, 2 or 3 minutes. Using tongs, rotate the peppers a quarter turn and continue cooking until blackened; continue turning and cooking until the pepper skins are charred all over.

3. Remove the peppers from the broiler to a medium-sized bowl. Cover with a plate or plastic wrap and set aside to cool, about 15 minutes.

4. Place a colander or sieve in another bowl. Holding a pepper over the colander to catch the seeds and skin fragments (and to allow the pepper juices to run through), peel the peppers. Dip your fingers in a bowl of water as you peel to rid them of burnt skin particles. Discard the charred skins and seeds.

5. Cut the roasted peppers into quarters and put them in a medium-sized bowl with the garlic, mint, oil, vinegar, and salt. If time allows, marinate at least 15 minutes, or even overnight.

6. To build the sandwiches: Using a toaster oven, warm the pita breads or split the English muffins and toast. Cut the pita breads in half and open the center pocket, or lay the bottoms of the English muffins on a work surface. Spread a layer of chèvre on the bread and add several leaves of mizuna or mesclun. Place one-quarter of each type of marinated pepper in the sandwiches. Sprinkle with salt and pepper, if desired. Close the sandwich and munch away! Place a pickle on each dish next to the sandwich.

Cooking Tip: The roasting of the peppers can be done ahead of time. Remove the cores and the charred skin and marinate the roasted peppers in a little vinegar and sea salt. (When peeling roasted peppers, keep a bowl of water handy to clean pieces of charred skin or seeds from your fingers.) Refrigerate until ready to use. They will last at least a week.

Nutritional Stars: Vitamin A, vitamin B3, vitamin B12, vitamin E, calcium, magnesium, zinc

Can You Top This?

Sauces and Toppings

Creamy Mushroom Sauce with Golden Garlic Bits

Yield: 3 cups   100% vegetarian

Chase away your PMS blues with this creamy and easy-to-make sauce over pasta.

PMS Benefits: The water-soluble B vitamins are easily excreted, especially when you are under stress. Mushrooms contain vitamin B5 and B vitamins that come to your rescue when you feel irritable and fatigued. High levels of vitamin B5 are also contained in eggs, whole grains, and seafood.

1 **8- to 10-ounce box button mushrooms, or any other favorite, washed**
1 **tablespoon extra-virgin olive oil or unsalted butter, preferably organic**
6 **cloves garlic, chopped coarsely**
1 **teaspoon herbal sea salt**
¼ **teaspoon ground white pepper**
1 **to 1½ cups purified water**
1 **cup cashew butter or tahini**

1. Slice the mushrooms thin and set aside.
2. In a large sauté pan, heat the olive oil or butter and add the garlic. Stir until the garlic begins to brown, about 2 minutes.
3. Add the mushrooms, herbal sea salt, pepper, and ½ cup water. Cover and bring to a boil. Lower flame to medium and cook 5 minutes.
4. In a medium-sized bowl or blender, whisk or blend the cashew butter with ½ cup water. Add more water, as needed, to make a thin sauce.
5. Stir the mushrooms and continue cooking uncovered, allowing some of the water to evaporate, about 5 minutes.
6. Pour the cashew sauce into the mushrooms and stir well. Continue heating until the sauce is warm. Do not boil. Pour over cooked soba or other whole grains.

Cooking Tip: When adding water to a nut or seed butter, pour in a little at a time and mix well. The gradual addition will keep the sauce from looking curdled. If it does happen, continue to add more water and stir—stir—stir.

Nutritional Stars: Vitamin B2, vitamin B3, vitamin B5, copper, magnesium, zinc

Sweet Red Pepper Butter

Yield: 2 cups   100% vegetarian

This creamy, sweet sauce is a summer treat when red peppers are in season and reasonably priced. Pour it over pasta or whole grains, spread over crackers, or ladle it over steamed vegetables.

PMS Benefits: Nonorganic peppers have a thin coating of wax that cannot be removed by washing. Disposing of this foreign material is a chore that stresses your system, adding to the load of environmental toxins and stresses your body must deal with every day. Choose organic peppers to please your body and prevent your PMS from flaring up.

> **4 red bell peppers**
> **2 tablespoons extra-virgin olive oil**
> **2 tablespoons flaxseed oil**
> **½ teaspoon herbal sea salt**
> **Pinch white pepper**
> **¼ cup homemade salt-free vegetable stock**

1. Position the broiler shelf about 3 inches from the heat source. Preheat the broiler.

2. Place the peppers on a nonglass baking tray. Roast under the broiler until the tops begin to char. Using tongs, rotate each pepper a quarter turn and continue this process until all sides have been charred.

3. Put the cooked peppers in a bowl and cover, or in a paper bag with the top closed. Set aside for 15 minutes. (This allows the peppers to cool and the skins to remoisten, so they are easier to peel.)

4. Place a sieve over a bowl. Peel the charred skins off the peppers, and remove the cores and seeds and discard.

5. In a blender or food processor, puree the peppers and juices with the oils, herbal sea salt, and pepper. Puree until very smooth. Add the stock and mix well. Use to top whole grains or pasta, as a spread on toast, or as a dip with breadsticks.

Cooking Tip: The roasting of the peppers can be done ahead of time. Remove the cores and the charred skin and marinate the roasted peppers in a little vinegar and sea salt. (When peeling roasted peppers, keep a bowl of water handy to clean pieces of charred skin or seeds from your fingers.) Refrigerate until ready to use. They will last at least a week.

Nutritional Stars: Vitamin A, vitamin B1, vitamin B6, vitamin C, omega-3 fatty acids

Chunky Onion-Celery Tomato Sauce

Yield: about 8 cups   100% vegetarian

Life without a rich, homemade tomato sauce just isn't possible!

PMS Benefits: The beta-carotenes found in bright red foods help to prevent acne associated with PMS.

3 tablespoons extra-virgin olive oil
6 cloves garlic, chopped
3 to 4 stalks celery, ends trimmed, chopped
2 onions, chopped
6 ripe beefsteak or 12 plum tomatoes, cores removed, chopped
   (see Note)
5 raisins or ½ carrot
2 bay leaves
2 teaspoons dried basil
1 to 2 teaspoons sea salt
½ teaspoon dried oregano
   Pinch dried sage or thyme
½ cup purified water (optional)
1 tablespoon unsalted butter, preferably organic

1. In a large saucepan, heat the olive oil and add the garlic, celery, and onions. Stir and sauté for 3 or 4 minutes.

2. Add the tomatoes, raisins or carrot, bay leaves, basil, 1 teaspoon salt, oregano, and sage or thyme. If the tomato mixture is very thick, add the water. Bring to a boil, covered. Lower heat and simmer for 30 to 40 minutes (fresh tomatoes need longer cooking). Stir occasionally.

3. Remove the bay leaves and stir in the butter. Taste and stir in additional salt, if needed. Serve hot on pasta or use in other dishes as suggested throughout the book. If you prefer, the sauce can be partly or completely pureed for a smoother texture.

Cooking Tip: Add raisins or a piece of carrot to a tomato sauce for additional sweetness—an extra that also tones down the acid taste of the tomatoes.

Note: The fresh tomatoes can be replaced with 1 box strained or 2 boxes crushed tomatoes or one 28-ounce can organic tomatoes (see Appendix for preferred brands).

Nutritional Stars: Vitamin A, vitamin B6, vitamin C, vitamin E, vitamin K, folic acid

Pumpkinseed and Garlic Romesco Sauce

Yield: 2 cups   100% vegetarian

Turn a bag of your favorite crunch nuts or seeds—almonds, walnuts, sunflower seeds, or pumpkinseeds—into this hearty sauce. It's also wonderful as a spread on whole-grain crackers.

PMS Benefits: Eating nuts and seeds is like taking a vitamin and mineral supplement. These tasty snacks have a wide range of important nutrients to quell the symptoms of PMS. Pumpkinseeds contain vitamin B2, iron, magnesium, and zinc, all of which help prevent PMS nervous tension.

1 **cup raw pumpkinseeds**
4 **cloves garlic, peeled**
4 **fresh plum tomatoes, cores removed, or 8 reconstituted sun-dried
     tomatoes, chopped**
½ **cup homemade salt-free vegetable stock or purified water**
½ **teaspoon herbal sea salt**
¼ **cup extra-virgin olive oil**
¼ **cup flaxseed oil**
   Ground pepper
2 **teaspoons cider vinegar**

1. In a medium-sized skillet, on moderate heat, dry-roast the pumpkinseeds and garlic. Cook until the seeds begin to pop and are lightly golden, about 5 minutes. Stir constantly to prevent burning.

2. Add the fresh or sun-dried tomatoes, stock or water, and herbal sea salt and stir. Lower flame and cover. Cook until the tomatoes soften, about 5 minutes. Turn off flame and let sit covered, 5 minutes.

3. In a blender or food processor, puree the pumpkinseed mixture until smooth. While the machine is running, drizzle in the oils. Add the pepper and vinegar, and mix well.

4. Using a rubber spatula, remove from the container to a beautiful ceramic serving bowl. Serve warm or at room temperature, as a crudité dip, over grains, or to season vegetables.

Cooking Tip: To dry-roast, use a heavy-bottomed skillet made of carbon steel, stainless steel, or cast iron. Avoid enamel cookware, since the enamel may chip when heated.

Nutritional Stars: Vitamin B2, copper, iron, magnesium, zinc

Fresh Mango-Papaya Sauce

Yield: 2½ cups   100% vegetarian

This tasty nutrient-rich fruit sauce is delicious over hot or cold cereal, pancakes, yogurt, toast, or served on the side with chicken or a fish fillet. It's so delicious you might even be tempted to eat it straight out of the saucepan!

PMS Benefits: Mangoes are especially high in vitamins B6, A, and E, which are among the most important nutrients for a woman with PMS. Try this mango sauce when you're craving sweet foods or feeling bloated.

> 2 **ripe mangoes**
> 1 **ripe papaya**
> 1½ **cups unsweetened apple juice**
>   **Pinch sea salt**
> 2 **tablespoons arrowroot or kuzu powder (see page 228)**
> 1 **teaspoon pure vanilla extract**
> 1 **to 2 tablespoons pure maple syrup or honey (optional)**

1. Place a mango on a plate to catch the juices while you are preparing it. Hold it upright and cut off slabs around the large interior pit. With a paring knife, score the flesh in a crosshatched pattern, being careful not to cut through the skin. With a spoon, scoop the mango into a bowl. Pour the juices into the bowl and repeat with the other mango. Discard the skin and pits.

2. Cut the papaya in half. With a spoon, remove and discard the dark seeds. Using a paring knife, score the flesh in a crosshatched pattern, being careful not to cut through the skin. With a spoon, scoop the papaya into the bowl with the mango. Discard the skin.

3. In a small saucepan, bring 1 cup juice to a boil with the salt.

4. In a small bowl, stir together the remaining ½ cup juice, arrowroot or kuzu, and vanilla. Pour the mixture into the hot apple juice; stir constantly until it thickens and clears. Cook another 30 seconds and turn off the flame.

5. Stir the cut fruit into the hot juice mixture, add the maple syrup, if using, and stir well. The sauce is now ready to pour over pancakes, yogurt, or sliced fresh fruit. Use warm or at room temperature.

Cooking Tip: For a change of color and taste, substitute other fruit for mangoes, for example, lime-green kiwi, orange persimmons, crimson strawberries, or midnight-blue blueberries.

Nutritional Stars: Vitamin A, vitamin B6, vitamin C, vitamin E

Desserts Are Good
for You!

Cookies and Cakes

A Fruit Dessert Sampling

Desserts to the PMS Rescue

Our dessert recipes offer you many sugar-free alternatives to satisfy a craving for sweets, which can be particularly strong at certain times of the month as hormone levels change. Sweeteners such as maple syrup and fruit juice do the trick without bringing on more symptoms.

But here is something we've noticed. When a woman has a craving for sweets and carbohydrates, she doesn't reach for a peach or an orange. It's cookies, pastry, or pie that's on her plate. So, we think there is another component to the menstrual sweet tooth—fat. The following recipes are designed to satisfy both needs, with nutritious sweets and top-quality fats.

Special Baking

Out of all the cooking methods suggested in this book, baking the whole-foods way will probably be the least familiar to you, but we assure you that it is as delicious and satisfying. For dry sugars we substitute liquid ones, such as maple syrup and honey. (See the Appendix for sweetness conversions.) This may change the consistency of your old and favorite recipes since this adds more liquid to the recipe. Whole-grain flours absorb a little more moisture than refined white flour, so to compensate for these two changes, reduce the liquid in the recipe by the amount of liquid sweetener added. The flour measurement can also be increased by half to the volume of liquid sweetener, if there is no other liquid to remove. If you substitute butter for margarine or vegetable shortening, the switch doesn't change how the batter behaves, and the volume amount of butter we add stays the same. Of course, what will change by baking with butter is the taste—and it's much better!

 ## Sesame Lemon Snaps with Almonds

Yield: 18 to 24 small cookies   100% vegetarian

Try these little cookie treats—topped with crunchy almonds and accented by the flavor of roasted sesame seeds and tangy lemon.

PMS Benefits: Sesame seeds contain calcium and magnesium, two minerals vital to the PMS menu. Calcium prevents painful cramps, and magnesium helps to control sugar cravings and stabilize moods.

(Sesame Lemon Snaps with Almonds—Continued)

1½ **cups rolled oatmeal (see Note)**
  2 **cups whole wheat pastry flour**
  ½ **cup unhulled sesame seeds**
  1 **teaspoon sea salt**
  ½ **teaspoon aluminum-free baking powder**
  ½ **cup unsalted butter, preferably organic, at room temperature**
  ¾ **cup pure maple syrup**
  ¼ **cup unsweetened apple juice, purified water, or plain yogurt**
      with active cultures
      Grated zest and juice of 3 lemons, preferably organic
  2 **teaspoons pure vanilla extract**
  1 **cup raw almonds**

1. Position the oven shelves so that the cookie sheets fit. Preheat the oven to 350 degrees. Line several cookie sheets with parchment paper or grease with additional butter.

2. In a blender or food processor, pulse-chop the oatmeal until partially ground. In a large bowl stir together the oatmeal, flour, sesame seeds, salt, and baking powder.

3. In another bowl or in the blender or food processor (without cleaning it from the oatmeal), cream the butter. Add the maple syrup, apple juice, water, or yogurt, lemon zest and juice, and vanilla. Cream together very well.

4. Combine the liquid and dry ingredients, stirring just until moistened.

5. Using two teaspoons (one to take up the batter and the other to push it off the spoon), drop by the spoonful onto the prepared cookie sheets. Press an almond into the center of each cookie.

6. Place in the oven and bake until golden, 8 to 12 minutes.

7. Remove the cookie trays from the oven. Using a metal spatula, transfer the cookies to a cooling rack. Once cool, store in a glass jar.

Cooking Tip: Take the butter out of the refrigerator before you start collecting the ingredients for your recipe. If you have forgotten to do this in time, place the butter in a dish on top of the preheating oven. Turn the butter over every few minutes, and it will soften quickly.

Note: Instead of the 2 cups oatmeal, add 1¾ cups more whole wheat pastry flour.

Nutritional Stars: Vitamin B2, vitamin B3, vitamin E, calcium, iron, magnesium

Walnut Oat Bars

Yield: 20 bars   100% vegetarian

Interested in eating desserts all day long? These bars are good enough to snack on at breakfast or during work.

PMS Benefits: Walnuts are a good source of omega-3 fatty acids, which help maintain vibrant skin and healthy, shiny hair, especially during your PMS days. Omega-3 is also found in flaxseeds and seafood, dark leafy greens, organ meats, and organic eggs.

- ½ **cup unsalted butter, preferably organic, at room temperature**
- ½ **cup pure maple syrup**
- ¼ **cup purified water or plain yogurt with active cultures (see Cooking Tip)**
- 2 **tablespoons unsulphured blackstrap molasses**
- 2 **teaspoons pure vanilla extract**
- ½ **teaspoon sea salt**
- 1½ **cups raw walnuts or Brazil nuts, chopped coarsely**
- 1 **cup rolled oatmeal**
- 1 **cup whole wheat pastry flour**
- ¼ **cup raw flaxseeds or sesame seeds**
- 1 **teaspoon aluminum-free baking powder**
- ½ **cup unsulphured currants or raisins**

1. Position the oven racks to fit a 9 × 9-inch baking pan. Preheat the oven to 350 degrees. Grease the pan with butter or line with parchment paper.

2. In a food processor or large bowl, cream the butter. Stir in the maple syrup, water or yogurt, molasses, vanilla, and salt and mix well.

3. In a medium-sized bowl, combine 1 cup walnuts with the oatmeal, flour, flaxseeds or sesame seeds, and baking powder. Add the currants or raisins, and stir again.

4. Combine the flour and butter mixtures, just until moistened.

5. With moistened hands, press the dough into the prepared baking pan. Sprinkle the remaining ½ cup walnuts over the top and press lightly into the dough.

6. Put in the oven and bake until golden, 15 to 20 minutes.

7. Remove from the oven. Set the pan on a cooling rack to cool for 10 to 15 minutes. While still warm, with a paring knife score the cake into bars.

8. Once cool, cut the bars all of the way through. (If parchment paper was used, lift the bars out of the pan and place on a cutting board first.) With a metal spatula, remove the bars to a plate for immediate munching or store in a glass jar.

(Walnut Oat Bars—Continued)

Cooking Tip: For the crunchiest bars, leave out the ¼ cup water or yogurt; for a more cakelike texture, add an additional ¼ cup.

Nutritional Stars: Vitamin B6, vitamin E, magnesium, omega-3 fatty acids

 # Apricot-Orange Corn Cake

Yield: 1 cake   100% vegetarian

Here is a cake kissed by the sweetness of springtime and with the heartiness of corn. We often use this recipe as a base for strawberry shortcake, made with real organic whipped cream!

PMS Benefits: Flavonoids include a group of compounds—citrin, hesperidin, rutin, and flavones—that modulate estrogen fluctuations by mimicking its structure and chemical activity. This process helps to ease anxiety, irritability, and mood swings. Citrus fruits, buckwheat, green peppers, as well as the apricots of this recipe, contain this nutrient.

- ½ **cup unsalted butter, preferably organic, at room temperature**
- ½ **cup pure maple syrup**
- 2 **eggs, preferably organic**
- ½ **cup all-fruit apricot or orange conserves**
  Grated zest and juice of 1 orange, preferably organic
- 2 **teaspoons pure vanilla extract**
- ¾ **teaspoon sea salt**
- 1 **cup high-lysine cornmeal or additional whole wheat pastry flour**
- 1 **cup whole wheat pastry flour**
- 1 **tablespoon aluminum-free baking powder**
- ½ **cup dried unsulphured apricots, chopped**
- ¼ **to ½ cup pumpkinseeds or sunflower seeds**

1. Position the oven shelves to fit a 9 × 9-inch baking pan. Preheat the oven to 350 degrees. Line the baking pan with parchment paper or grease the pan with additional butter.

2. In a food processor or large bowl, cream the butter. Beat in the maple syrup, eggs, apricot or orange conserves, orange zest and juice, vanilla, and salt. Mix well.

3. In a medium-sized bowl, combine the cornmeal and wheat flour, baking powder, and apricots.

4. Combine the butter and flour mixtures. Stir until just moistened.

5. Pour the batter into the prepared baking pan. Top with pumpkinseeds or sunflower seeds, using as many or as few as you desire. Place in the oven and bake until golden brown, 25 to 30 minutes.

6. Remove the cake from the oven and place the pan on a cooling rack. Once cool, cut the cake into squares or wedges. Store covered.

Cooking Tip: Turn a cake recipe into muffins by spooning the batter into paper-lined muffin cups and bake until golden on top, about half the cake-baking time.

Nutritional Stars: Flavonoids, calcium, magnesium, zinc

White Fig and Pear Upside-down Ginger Cake with Maple-roasted Pecans

Yield: 1 cake   100% vegetarian

We find this crunchy, fruity cake to be a hit with company, but don't wait for friends to show up to bake it.

PMS Benefits: Heavy menstrual flow leads to loss of iron and persistent fatigue. Reverse PMS exhaustion by eating iron-rich figs and pears. Other reliable sources of iron are blackstrap molasses, seaweed, beans, and raisins.

- ¾ **cup unsalted butter, preferably organic, at room temperature**
- 1 **cup raw pecan or walnut halves**
- 1 **cup pure maple syrup**
- ¼ **cup unsulphured blackstrap molasses**
- 1 **teaspoon powdered ginger**
- 1 **teaspoon sea salt**
- 1 **cup unsulphured dried white figs, cherries, prunes, or raisins**
- 4 **bosc pears, cored and quartered**
- ½ **cup rice, almond, or other milk**
- 2 **teaspoons pure vanilla extract**
- 1 **egg, preferably organic**
- 1¼ **cups whole wheat pastry flour**
- 2 **teaspoons aluminum-free baking powder**
- 1 **teaspoon cinnamon**
- ¼ **teaspoon powdered cloves**

(White Fig and Pear Upside-down Ginger Cake with Maple-roasted Pecans—Continued)

1. Position the oven shelves to fit a 9 × 9-inch square baking pan or a 9- or 10-inch-deep pie plate. Preheat the oven to 350 degrees. Line the pan with parchment paper and lightly butter, or omit paper and grease thickly with additional butter.

2. In a blender or food processor, grind ¼ cup pecans or walnuts. Dust the bottom of the buttered pan with the ground nuts, pressing them into the buttered bottom.

3. In a small saucepan, melt ¼ cup butter. Mix in ½ cup maple syrup, the molasses, ginger, and ½ teaspoon salt. Stir in the remaining ¾ cup pecans or walnuts.

4. Remove the stem of the figs, and cut them in half, lengthwise. Lay the figs on top of the ground nuts, cut side down. Using a slotted spoon, lift the pecans or walnuts from the maple mixture. Spread them in a layer on top of the figs. Lay the pears across the nuts. Drizzle the remaining maple mixture on top.

5. In a medium-sized bowl, cream the remaining ½ cup butter. Mix in the remaining ½ cup maple syrup, the milk, vanilla, egg, and remaining ½ teaspoon salt.

6. In another bowl mix the flour, baking powder, cinnamon, and cloves. Combine the liquid and dry ingredients, stirring until just moistened. Pour the batter over the pears. Place the pan in the oven and bake until the top is golden and the cake begins to pull away from the sides, 40 to 50 minutes.

7. Remove the cake from the oven and place on a metal cooling rack. Once cool, slide a knife blade around the edges of the pan to loosen the cake. Place a serving platter on top of the cake pan and, holding both firmly, turn them upside down. Lift off the baking pan. (You may need to tap the bottom of the cake pan with a wooden spoon to loosen further.) If the pan was prepared with parchment paper, peel it off and discard. Cut the cake into squares or wedges.

Cooking Tip: Free-range chickens produce organic eggs that are far more flavorful than the average egg. Yolks are bright yellow-orange, shells are thick, and since organic eggs are usually fresher, whites stay close to the yolk when opened.

Nutritional Stars: B-complex vitamins, calcium, iron, magnesium, zinc

Silky Peach Custard with Pistachios and Cardamom Swirl

Yield: 4 to 6 servings   100% vegetarian

Add some sweetness to your peaches by pureeing them with fruit juice and swirling in a little almond butter.

PMS Benefits: Niacin aids in blood circulation and healthy skin. Without enough of this B vitamin, such PMS symptoms as fatigue, depression, headaches, insomnia, and acne may occur. You will find ample amounts of niacin in many foods, including peaches, avocados, pinto and black beans, whole grains, and mushrooms.

¼ **ounce gelatin (1 package) or 1 bar agar**
2 **cups unsweetened apple-peach juice**
2 **ripe peaches, pitted and quartered**
½ **cup plus 2 tablespoons all-fruit peach conserves**
¼ **cup pure maple syrup**
3 **tablespoons arrowroot or kuzu powder (see page 228)**
   Pinch sea salt
2 **teaspoons pure vanilla extract**
¼ **cup roasted, unsalted pistachios, shelled and chopped coarsely**
1 **teaspoon powdered cardamom or cinnamon**
2 **tablespoons raw almond or cashew butter**
4 **to 6 fresh strawberries or ½ pint raspberries**

1. In a medium-sized saucepan, dissolve the gelatin or agar in 1 cup juice. Heat over a low flame to further dissolve, about 3 minutes.

2. In a blender or food processor, puree the peaches in the remaining 1 cup juice. Add ½ cup conserves with the maple syrup, arrowroot or kuzu, and salt. Blend again. While stirring with a whisk, pour the peach mixture into the saucepan. Increase the heat and bring to a boil, stirring continuously. Once it is boiling, stir with a wooden spoon. The mixture will begin to thicken and clear.

3. Stir in the vanilla and cook another 30 seconds. Pour the hot mixture into a shallow, nonmetal baking pan or large bowl. Set aside to cool and firm, or refrigerate for 1 hour.

4. In a small bowl, mix the pistachios, cardamom or cinnamon, and the remaining 2 tablespoons conserves. Set aside.

5. Once set, using a blender or food processor, puree the pudding with the almond or cashew butter. Spoon into individual parfait glasses or wine goblets. Add 1½ tablespoons of the pistachio mixture to each glass. Using a butter knife, swirl the

(Silky Peach Custard with Pistachios and Cardamom Swirl—Continued)

mixture into the pudding. Top each with a strawberry or a spoonful of raspberries, and enjoy the fruit of your labors!

Cooking Tip: Pure vanilla extract is made from freshly harvested vanilla beans that have been aged in alcohol at least three months. You can make your own by splitting three vanilla beans and slipping them into a pint bottle of bourbon or vodka.

Nutritional Stars: Vitamin B2, vitamin B3, vitamin E, calcium, iron

 # The Best Peach 'n Apple Open-faced Pie

Yield: 1 pie   100% vegetarian

Prepared with or without a crust, this pie tastes luscious. Top this treat with a quick sprinkle of unsweetened coconut and nuts to give it a rich taste and satisfy your sweet tooth in a healthy way.

PMS Benefits: Whole wheat flour and white flour are not at all the same. When a grain is refined, the bran and germ are removed, and the central core of the grain, called the endosperm, is retained. Bran contains fiber and many B vitamins, and the germ is full of healthy oils, vitamin E, and other nutrients. The core of the grain is mostly starch. All parts of the grain are needed to provide the many nutrients the body requires, but white flour only delivers a small percentage.

4 peaches, cut in half, pitted, and sliced
3 apples, quartered, cored, and sliced
½ cup unsulphured raisins
¼ cup unsulphured dried apricots, chopped or sliced
¼ to ½ cup pure maple syrup plus additional as needed
2 tablespoons arrowroot (see page 225) or fine tapioca
2 teaspoons cinnamon
1 teaspoon powdered ginger
Grated zest and juice of 1 lemon, preferably organic
2 pinches sea salt
1 prepared whole-grain pie crust, unbaked (see Note)
4 tablespoons unsalted butter, preferably organic
½ cup raw walnuts or almonds, chopped coarsely
½ cup raw pecans, chopped coarsely

1. Position the oven shelves so that a pie pan fits in the center. Preheat the oven to 350 degrees.

2. In a large bowl, combine the peaches, apples, raisins, apricots, ¼ cup maple syrup, arrowroot or tapioca, cinnamon, ginger, lemon zest and juice, and salt. Stir well. Taste the fruit to determine sweetness, and if needed, add the remaining ¼ cup maple syrup. Stir again.

3. Pour the fruit into the pie crust and dot with small pieces of butter.

4. In a small bowl, combine the walnuts or almonds, pecans, and 2 to 3 tablespoons maple syrup. Top the pie with the nut mixture. Put the filled pie on a baking sheet and place in the preheated oven. Bake until the fruit is tender and the nuts are lightly golden and roasted, about 45 minutes.

5. Remove the baked pie from the oven to a metal cooling rack to cool and set for at least 10 minutes before cutting.

Cooking Tip: The zest of a citrus fruit is the outer layer of color that tops the white layer known as the pith. Avoid the chemicals sprayed on the surface of the fruits by purchasing organic fruit. You can also find organic bottled zest in the natural-food store.

Note: Prepare this pie without the crust by placing the fruit in a greased baking pan.

Nutritional Stars: Vitamin A, B-complex vitamins, flavonoids, calcium, magnesium, zinc

 ## Cathy's Easy Fresh-fruit Salad

Yield: 4 servings   100% vegetarian

Fruit salad is a simple pleasure and a great finger food for kids. Snack on the handy slices of apples and pears, or on blueberries, strawberries, and more.

PMS Benefits: Potassium alleviates PMS irritability and maintains proper blood-pressure levels. Banana, kiwi, apricots, beans, and sweet potatoes are rich in this mineral. They also contain lignins, a type of phytohormone that helps modulate estrogen. This helps prevent menstrual mood swings associated with a dominance of either estrogen or progesterone. Flaxseeds contain one hundred times more lignins than any other plant studied.

    1 **to 2 clementine oranges or mandarin tangerines**
    1 **ripe banana, peeled**
    1 **kiwi, peeled**
    1 **apple of choice, preferably organic, quartered and core removed**
    1 **tablespoon unsweetened coconut**
    ½ **cup unsweetened apple juice (optional)**

(Cathy's Easy Fresh-fruit Salad—Continued)

1. Peel and separate the clementines or tangerines into individual sections. Place in a medium-sized bowl.

2. Cut the banana and kiwi into small pieces and add to the bowl. If the apple is organic, chop three of the quarters into small pieces; otherwise, peel the apple before chopping. Add to the other fruit with the coconut and toss. Place in a serving bowl.

3. Cut the remaining apple quarter into thin slivers. Fan the slivers out on top of the fruit as a garnish and serve. (If the fruit is going to be stored before serving or if there is any left over, add the juice to keep the fruit from turning brown.)

Cooking Tip: To peel a kiwi, cut it in half around the diameter. Scoop out its flesh with a small spoon, leaving the skin behind.

Nutritional Stars: Vitamin B6, vitamin C, flavonoids, folic acid, calcium, potassium

---

PMS Fruit Salad Nutrients

- Apples: fiber—prevents hormone imbalance
- Apricots: vitamin A, flavonoids—help lessen menstrual flow
- Banana: vitamin B6—counteracts sugar cravings
- Blueberries, raspberries: flavonoids—steady mood swings
- Cantaloupe: vitamin A—reduces abdominal bloating
- Citrus: flavonoids—lessen cramping
- Figs: calcium, magnesium—promote restful sleep, reduce irritability
- Kiwi: vitamin C—combats stress
- Mango: vitamins A, E, B6—reduce breast tenderness and fluid retention
- Papaya: vitamins C, A—help prevent anemia, fatigue, and painful menstrual cramps
- Pears: iron—prevents anemia
- Strawberries: vitamin C, folic acid—reduce heavy menstrual bleeding and irritability

Fresh Blueberry Marzipan Tart
with Orange Glaze

Yield: 1 tart   100% vegetarian

This tart is a beauty, full of luscious fresh blueberries—and easy to make. You won't even miss the refined sugar!

PMS Benefits: Almonds are a good source of protein and are high in heart-friendly monounsaturated fats, the same as those found in olive oil. They are also high in vitamin E, an important nutrient that reduces the likelihood of PMS symptoms such as irritability, anxiety, and depression.

- 2 **teaspoons plus 2 tablespoons unsalted butter, preferably organic, at room temperature**
- 2 **tablespoons whole-grain flour**
- 2½ **cups raw almonds**
- 5 **eggs, preferably organic**
- ⅔ **cup pure maple syrup**
- 1 **teaspoon pure almond extract**
- **Pinch sea salt**
- 1 **cup unsweetened apple juice**
- 4 **tablespoons all-fruit orange, apricot, or peach conserves**
- **Grated zest and juice of 2 oranges, preferably organic**
- 2 **tablespoons arrowroot or kuzu powder (see page 228)**
- 2 **pints blueberries, washed and dried (see Cooking Tip)**
- **Cream, freshly whipped, preferably organic (optional)**

1. Position the oven shelves so that an 8- or 9-inch springform pan fits in the center. Preheat the oven to 350 degrees. Prepare the springform pan by greasing the entire pan—both bottom and sides—with 2 teaspoons butter, and dust with flour. Tap the pan, upside down and over the sink, to remove any excess flour.

2. In a blender or food processor, grind the almonds to a fine powder. Add the eggs, maple syrup, almond extract, and salt. Blend until very smooth.

3. Pour the batter into the springform pan and place on a baking sheet. Bake in the oven until the top is firm to the touch and golden, about 20 minutes. Remove from the oven and place on a metal rack to cool.

4. In a small saucepan, simmer ¾ cup apple juice until reduced to ½ cup.

5. Add 2 tablespoons conserves, the remaining 2 tablespoons butter, and the orange zest and juice. Stir until dissolved.

(Fresh Blueberry Marzipan Tart with Orange Glaze—Continued)

6. Dilute the arrowroot or kuzu in the remaining ¼ cup apple juice. Add to the saucepan and cook until clear; cook 30 seconds more, stirring constantly.

7. Spread the remaining 2 tablespoons of conserves on top of the marzipan cake in a thin layer. Spread the blueberries over the conserves. Spoon the hot glaze on the blueberries, being sure to cover them all. Set aside to cool.

8. Serve with freshly whipped cream, if desired.

Cooking Tip: To wash berries, fill a bowl with purified water. Add the berries and remove any floating stems and leaves. With your hands, remove the berries from the water to a colander. Pick through each handful and remove any stems. (For strawberries, use a paring knife or strawberry picker to remove the green leaves.) Dry the drained berries on a cotton cloth spread on the counter.

Nutritional Stars: Vitamin A, vitamin B2, vitamin B3, vitamin C, vitamin E, flavonoids, calcium, iron, magnesium, omega-3 fatty acids

 ## Apple, Prune, and Walnut Cobbler

Yield: 6 to 8 servings   100% vegetarian

This dessert of baked fruit topped by a light and nutty cake provides a daily dose of PMS nutrients.

PMS Benefits: Unless you've been diagnosed with iron-deficiency anemia, it is best not to supplement with iron, which can be toxic in high amounts. We recommend iron-rich foods, such as prunes and raisins, seafood, whole grains, beans, and blackstrap molasses, as part of your daily intake. These foods will also keep your blood sugar steady and PMS symptoms down to a minimum.

- 2 teaspoons plus ¼ cup unsalted butter, preferably organic, at room temperature
- 6 apples, preferably organic, cored and sliced (see Note)
- ¾ cup pure maple syrup
- 2 teaspoons cinnamon
- ½ teaspoon nutmeg
- ½ teaspoon ginger powder
- ¼ teaspoon sea salt plus additional as needed
- 3 teaspoons arrowroot (see page 225)
- 1 tablespoon lemon juice
- 1 cup rice or almond milk, or plain yogurt with active cultures

2 **teaspoons pure vanilla extract**
1 **cup whole wheat pastry flour**
2 **teaspoons aluminum-free baking powder**
½ **cup raw walnuts or pecans**
   Cream, freshly whipped, preferably organic, or yogurt (optional)

1. Position the oven shelves so that a 13 × 9 × 2-inch rectangular baking pan fits in the center. Preheat the oven to 350 degrees. Grease the pan with 2 teaspoons butter.

2. In a large bowl, combine the apples, ½ cup maple syrup, 1 teaspoon cinnamon, the nutmeg, ginger, a pinch of salt, the arrowroot, and lemon juice. Pour into the prepared pan.

3. In a small saucepan, melt ¼ cup butter. Add the remaining ¼ cup maple syrup, rice or almond milk, and vanilla. In a medium-sized bowl, combine the flour, ¼ teaspoon salt, baking powder, and remaining cinnamon. Mix the liquid and dry ingredients together—it will be a runny batter.

4. Drizzle the batter over the apples and top with the walnuts or pecans. Put in the oven and bake until the fruit is tender, the nuts are roasted, and the top is golden brown—30 to 40 minutes.

5. Serve warm with a spoonful of freshly whipped cream or a dollop of yogurt, if desired.

Cooking Tip: The skins of organic apples add fiber and color to your dessert. If you choose nonorganic apples, make sure to peel them in order to remove their wax coating.

Note: Other fresh fruits, such as peaches, pears, blueberries, or cherries, can be substituted for or mixed with the apples.

Nutritional Stars: B-complex vitamins, calcium, magnesium, iron, zinc, omega-3 fatty acids

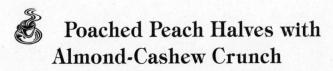

Poached Peach Halves with Almond-Cashew Crunch

Yield: 4 servings   100% vegetarian

Use any fresh fruit in season to create a nourishing and soothing dessert that is also good as a breakfast food or a quick snack.

PMS Benefits: Peaches contain higher amounts of iron, riboflavin, and niacin than most other fruits. These needed nutrients are important to maintain healthy blood and resilient nerves throughout the month.

(Poached Peach Halves with Almond-Cashew Crunch—Continued)

- **4 peaches, cut in half and pitted (see Cooking Tip)**
- **1 cup unsweetened apple juice**
- **Grated zest and juice of 1 lemon, preferably organic**
- **¼ teaspoon plus a pinch sea salt**
- **1 cup raw almonds**
- **1 cup raw cashews**
- **¼ cup unsalted butter, preferably organic**
- **¼ cup pure maple syrup**
- **1 tablespoon unsulphured blackstrap molasses**
- **1 teaspoon cinnamon**

1. In a medium-sized saucepan, combine the peaches, apple juice, lemon zest and juice, and pinch salt. Bring to a boil, covered, lower heat, and simmer until tender when a fork is inserted, 10 to 12 minutes.

2. Position the oven rack so that a baking sheet fits in the middle. Preheat the oven to 350 degrees. Prepare a baking sheet with parchment paper.

3. Put the almonds and cashews into a medium-sized bowl.

4. In a small saucepan, heat the butter, maple syrup, molasses, cinnamon, and ¼ teaspoon salt. Pour over the nuts and stir well. Spread on the baking sheet in a thin layer. Put in the preheated oven and bake until the nuts are roasted, about 15 minutes. Remove from the oven and cool thoroughly.

5. Serve the peaches in individual bowls. Break the crunch into pieces and spoon on top of the peaches. Serve warm.

Cooking Tip: Choose peaches that are slightly underripe and still firm. Once baked they will soften and sweeten from the cooking process.

Nutritional Stars: Vitamin B2, vitamin B3, vitamin E, copper, magnesium, iron, riboflavin, niacin

APPENDIX

Understanding and Knowing Your Ingredients

Agar: A vegetarian source of gelatin that is used commercially as a stabilizer, thickener, binding agent, and emulsifier. Most coastal areas have used agar and other derivatives of sea plants for centuries. It is available in bars, flakes, or powder. Agar can be substituted for gelatin but has stronger setting properties, so less of it is required. To get 2½ cups liquid use ¼ cup flakes, 1 bar, or 2 teaspoons powder. Also see "Seaweeds" and "Gelatin."

Almond butter: See "Nut and seed butters."

Anchovies: Small, silvery fish from the Mediterranean and southern European coastlines. They are generally filleted, salt-cured, and canned in oil. They can also be found packed in coarse salt. To reduce their salt content, soak them in purified water for 20 to 30 minutes, then drain and pat with paper toweling. Use sparingly.

Arrowroot: A powder made from the cassava plant, which Native Americans used to draw out poisons from arrow wounds—thus the name. It thickens at low temperatures, is easy to digest, contains trace minerals, and when used turns liquids into translucent and shiny sauces. When using in place of flour, use half the amount of arrowroot. Dissolve it in cold water and stir into the liquid at the end of the cooking period. Return to a boil, and as the liquid turns clear, cook another 30 seconds. Also see "Kuzu."

Bacon and cured meats: Used occasionally, this "treat" food is wonderful for adding flavor to a dish. Commercial bacon and cured meats are processed with sodium nitrite or nitrate food additives used to stabilize the pink or red color in meats, enhance flavor, and protect against bacterial growth. When heated, nitrites react chemically with amine compounds to form nitrosamines, which can be carcinogenic. This type of bacon also contains BHT (a preservative), various sugars (white, brown, and/or corn syrup), and an excessive amount of salt. If bacon or cured meats are used, we recommend the kind without chemicals and preservatives, found in natural-food markets.

Beans: Beans are low in fat and contain only 125 calories per ½ cup serving. They are also high in fiber that helps eliminate excess estrogen and ease menstrual woes. Beans are also a valuable source of protein—½ cup of cooked beans contains the same amount of protein as an 1½ ounces of ground beef, about 7 grams. (Three to four ounces of meat is the recommended average serving size.) Plus beans supply B vitamins that help a woman manage stress, which can be especially hard to tolerate premenstrually. Finally, beans are high in magnesium, which helps lessen the inflammation associated with breast tenderness.

Black beans, fermented: An Asian flavoring prepared by preserving black beans in brine and then drying them. Their flavor is quite delicate, and not very salty.

Bread crumbs, whole-grain: These are missing the hydrogenated fats, chemical flavorings, and preservatives and contain the fiber, B vitamins, and minerals of whole grains. They are available in the natural-food store, or you can make your own by pulverizing stale or toasted whole-grain bread, crackers, or breadsticks in a blender or food processor. Store extras in the freezer or refrigerator.

Brown rice: According to the "Composition of Foods," published by the USDA, when brown rice is compared with white, brown has 12% more protein, 33% more calcium, five times more vitamin B1, 67% more vitamin B2, three times more niacin, and two and a half times as much potassium and iron. It has 100% more vitamin E, as there is none left in white rice.

Butter: See "Friendly Fats," page 232.

Buttermilk: A tangy yogurtlike fermented milk with living cultures that are beneficial to digestion and assimilation. It is thicker than milk and lower in fat. Also see "Yogurt."

Conserves: Naturally sweetened all-fruit jams made from good-quality fruit of optimum ripeness, without any added sweetener. Spreads and butters such as peach spread and apple butter can also be made without adding refined sugars. By law, "preserves" must contain sugar.

Cornmeal, high-lysine: High-lysine cornmeal contains the amino acid lysine that is missing in commercial cornmeal. This hybrid strain maintains its sweet and nutty taste for a longer time, keeping the cornmeal from going rancid and tasting bitter. Store in the refrigerator or freezer.

Dehydrated vegetables: Garlic and onion are the most common in this category, and are found as flakes and powdered. If using the fresh ones takes too much prep time, these can add plenty of flavor to the recipes. Look for those without additives or preservatives. Also see "Herbs and spices."

Eggs: Eggs provide a good source of high-quality protein, plus iron, zinc, and vitamins A, B2, D, E, and K.

Eggs, organic: The chickens that lay these eggs are free of antibiotics and added hormones that can burden your system. When chickens are free-range, they eat a more natural diet, and their eggs tend to have thicker shells, bright yellow-orange yolks, and a richer flavor. These are the eggs we recommend you use.

Flour, whole wheat: There are two whole wheat flours available. One is whole wheat pastry flour, ground from soft wheat and best used for cookies, cakes, quick breads, pancakes, and other pastries. The other is whole wheat flour that is derived from hard wheat, best used for yeast or sourdough breads. These flours can be used interchangeably when called for in a roux, sauce, or to coat vegetables or meat. Most other grains are available in flour form and they can be experimented with for taste and texture preferences.

Gelatin: An odorless, tasteless, and colorless jelling agent. It is a pure protein derived from beef and veal bones, cartilage, and other tissues. Granulated gelatin is the most common form of unsweetened commercial gelatin on the market. It comes in boxes of $\frac{1}{4}$-ounce envelopes, each of which will jell 2 cups of liquid. Soak it first in cold liquid for 3 to 5 minutes to soften the granules so they will dissolve evenly when heated. Also see "Agar."

Ghee: This is butter that has been clarified to remove the milk solids. It can be cooked on a higher flame than butter or oil without smoking. Organic ghee is available premade or you can make your own. To make ghee: In a small saucepan, over low heat, melt $\frac{1}{2}$ pound unsalted organic butter. Remove from the heat and cool for a few minutes. Place in the refrigerator or freezer until hardened. Skim the thin layer of foam from the top and discard. Using a spoon, scoop the clarified butter into a small glass container. Discard the remaining milk solids. Store at room temperature. It will last for 4 to 6 months. Also see "Friendly Fats," page 232.

Grains: See "The Whole-Grain and Pasta Story," page 83.

Grains, cream of: Finely ground cereals made from whole grains such as wheat, rye, rice, corn (grits), or buckwheat that cook in 5 minutes. They make excellent breakfast cereals.

Heat diffuser: A round metal utensil that is placed between the pot and the flame to spread the flame and keep a thin-bottomed pot from burning.

Herbal sea salt: A combination of light and flavorful herbs that is added to sea salt. Look for brands without hydrolyzed vegetable protein, hydrogenated oils, sugar, monosodium glutamate (MSG), preservatives, or free-flowing chemicals. Herbal sea salt is a little less salty than sea salt alone, and can be used interchangeably. You'll also open fewer herb and spice bottles to achieve rich flavors. Also see "Brands We Trust," page 238.

Herbs and spices: Not all herbs and spices are bottled in the same way. Commercial herbs and spices are frequently mixed with preservatives to maintain freshness. We prefer the varieties without these additives. Many organically grown herbs and spices are now available. Also see "Dehydrated Vegetables."

Jícama: A fleshy tuber from Mexico, with a light-brown skin. It can be used raw, in salads, or as a crudité; also sautéed, boiled, or steamed. Peel the outer skin before using. Raw, it has a sweet taste and a texture similar to an apple; after cooking, it still stays crisp.

Juice, bottled: We recommend unsweetened juice that is one hundred percent fruit juice, and is unfiltered, and without preservatives or refined sugars. These juices are usually cloudy, and contain some fiber and pectin; they have more nutrients than the clear varieties. Many commercial juices are made from fruit purees, concentrates, or nectars, which have added water and/or sugars. If the juice is labeled drink, cocktail, or punch, it contains very little fruit juice and a great deal of sugar, artificial flavors, and colorings.

Kasha: Kasha is dry-roasted buckwheat that is available in whole, fine, medium, and coarse grains. The unmilled whole-grain triangular-shaped kernels are the ones we prefer and are the best-tasting. Unroasted buckwheat is a creamy white color;

once roasted, it is brown. Since it is pretoasted, this grain does not get washed before cooking, and takes 10 minutes to cook.

Kohlrabi: A cruciferous vegetable in the family with cabbages, cauliflower, broccoli, and Brussels sprouts. The root has a delicate turnip flavor and can be added to stews, soups, or used as a crudité. The green tops can be simmered, steamed, stir-fried, or served raw in salads.

Kuzu: The powdered root of the kudzu plant, which when dry looks like small, white rocks. It has thickening properties similar to those of arrowroot and also medicinal effects. In the Orient, it is used for nausea, colds, indigestion, and to help treat diarrhea. It must be dissolved in cold water before being cooked. Once it thickens, it has a bright sheen and sparkle that is unique to kuzu. It can give the texture of pudding or gravy, depending on how much is used to thicken a liquid. To substitute for arrowroot, use half the amount of kuzu; when substituting for flour, use a quarter of the amount.

Lemon and lime juice: Fresh citrus juices taste best and have lots of vitamin C. Bottled juices are a great convenience and can save labor when a recipe requires a quantity of citrus juice. There are several bottled brands without preservatives and other chemicals, and they can now be found organic, too. See "Brands We Trust," page 238.

Liver, organic: A wide range of vitamins and minerals are contained in this organ meat, including vitamins A, K, and B12, folic acid, niacin, selenium, zinc, and iron. Liver from an animal raised on clean feed, which hasn't been given antibiotics or supplemental hormones, and has had minimal environmental contamination is what we recommend. If organic is not available—skip the liver.

Maple syrup: Pure maple syrup is the sap of the maple tree, boiled until the water has evaporated and the maple sugars have concentrated. It is not at all the same as maple-flavored syrup, which is produced from less expensive sugars, such as corn syrup, with artificial maple flavor and coloring added. Pure maple syrup has many minerals, including calcium, potassium, manganese, magnesium, phosphorus, and iron.

Milk substitutes: To replace cow's milk in a recipe, rice, oat, and soy milks are available.

Miso: A fermented bean paste with a living, active culture, traditionally made from cooked soybeans and/or other beans and grains, and sea salt and water. Use miso in soups or sauces instead of bouillon or dilute with water for stock; when using miso in a recipe, reduce the salt. It can also be used instead of salt in salad dressing and sauce, or to flavor beans, grains, or stew. The taste is similar to soy sauce but lighter. We prefer the sweet taste of chickpea miso, which is also lower in salt.

Mushrooms: Available both dried and fresh, they are a delight for both their taste and their nutrients. Mushrooms can be added to almost any dish. Soak **dry mushrooms** in purified water for 15 to 20 minutes. Squeeze excess water from them and cook. **Fresh mushrooms** need a quick rinse in water to remove any peat moss left from the growing and packaging process. Do not soak fresh mushrooms in water or their flavor will dilute.

Button mushrooms are cultivated white mushrooms with a mild and earthy flavor.
Cepes (also known as porcini) have a nutty favor and strong mushroom taste.
Chanterelles are known for their apricotlike aroma and taste.
Enoki have a long, thin stem with a tiny snow-white cap. They are very mild-tasting and have an appealing crunchy texture.
Morels have a rich, smoky, nutty, and woodsy flavor. Dried morels are more intense-tasting than fresh ones.
Oyster mushrooms have a robust flavor with a slightly peppery taste that dissipates when cooked.
Portobello is a large dark-brown mushroom and when sautéed, it has a robust and meaty taste and texture.
Shiitake have a distinct aroma and taste. The dried ones have a chewy texture, while the fresh shiitake are milder in both taste and texture. The stems are best when used in a stock and then discarded.
Tree ear or *cloud ear mushrooms* are available in dried form and expand five to six times after soaking. They impart little flavor, but add a springy texture.

Nut and seed butters: Raw or lightly roasted nuts and seeds that are ground to the consistency of paste. Store in the refrigerator, and use in a timely fashion.

Oils: See "Friendly Fats," page 232.

Parchment paper: Eliminates the need to grease baking pans and pie plates. Please see "Brands We Trust," page 238.

Pasta: See "Whole-wheat pasta," "Soba noodles," "Udon noodles," and "The Whole-Grain and Pasta Story," page 83.

Pasta, flavored: Artichoke, spinach, tomato, squid ink, etc.—these are all made with a base of refined white or semolina flour, which have had many of the nutrients and fiber removed. These are inferior to whole-grain pastas, and it is best for you to leave them alone.

Pasta, whole-grain: Use whole-grain pastas made with whole wheat, brown-rice, corn, or buckwheat flours. See "Whole-wheat pasta," "Soba noodles," "Udon noodles," and "The Whole-Grain and Pasta Story," page 83.

Purified water: See "Water and Purification Systems," page 243.

Salad dressing: Bottled dressings and dips are full of sugar, salt, refined oils, chemicals, and preservatives. Look for brands that use better-quality oils, such as extra-virgin olive oil, and that are made without refined sugars, chemicals, or preservatives. (Add a few tablespoons of water to dips and you have created a creamy and delicious salad dressing.)

Salt, common: Table salt is manufactured by using steam heat under pressure of up to 1,200 degrees and then flash-cooling to produce crystals. Aluminum is then added to this salt to prevent caking; potassium iodide is added to provide iodine, important for thyroid function in people who don't eat fish regularly; a sugar (dextrose) to hold the molecules of iodine in the salt; a whitening agent, sodium bicarbonate, to offset the tendency of potassium iodide to turn the salt purple; plus various anticaking agents such as sodium silico-aluminate, sodium ferro-cyanide, and yellow prussiate of soda. We do not recommend this type of salt.

Salt, sea: This salt is produced by the solar evaporation of seawater and has no chemical additives, sugar, or aluminum. It is only about seventy-eight percent sodium chloride and contains many trace minerals. This is the only salt we recommend.

Seaweeds: A rich source of easy-to-digest proteins, vitamins (A, B, B12, C, and E), and minerals (calcium, phosphorous, magnesium, iron, and iodine). Included in this category is dulse, kelp, and kombu. Also see "Agar."

Soba noodles: Made from one hundred percent buckwheat flour or a mixture of buckwheat and wheat flours, soba can be served chilled or hot. The shape is similar to spaghetti, although soba noodles taste nothing like it. Soba is better with nontomato sauces, such as our Creamy Mushroom Sauce with Golden Garlic Bits. Also see "Whole-wheat pasta," "Udon noodles," and "The Whole-Grain and Pasta Story," page 83.

Soy sauce: Good-quality soy sauce is naturally brewed in wooden kegs for months and is made with water, soy beans, sea salt, and sometimes wheat. The imported and natural soy sauces may be labeled as real soy sauce, tamari, or shoyu. These are the types we recommend. The commercially produced product is made from refined soy meal, which is treated with hydrochloric acid and then heated. Next, sodium carbonate is added to neutralize the acid. This type has additives including caramel color, corn syrup, BHT, and other preservatives, and has never been fermented. We suggest you never use this kind of soy sauce.

Spices: See "Herbs and spices."

Sugar, white: A highly refined product made from sugar cane or sugar beets. During processing, fiber, vitamins, minerals, amino acids, and trace elements are removed. Since refined sugar is lacking fiber, it is absorbed into the bloodstream very quickly, causing the pancreas and adrenal glands to overreact. This can lead to irritability, bloating, and fatigue. Refined white sugar contains no nutrients other than simple carbohydrates, but requires some vitamins and minerals to be metabolized. Therefore, it takes nutrients away from the body's other needs, such as cell growth, and protein synthesis. Women with PMS cannot afford to lose any vitamins or minerals, all of which are needed to maintain hormonal balance, steady blood sugar, and a healthy nervous system. It is recommended that you avoid sugar and products containing it. Also see "Maple syrup."

Tahini: A very versatile ground sesame paste that has the amino acids to complement grains, as it is rich in methionine and low in lysine. It is suitable to use tahini on toast, in puddings, spreads, dips, salad dressings, soups, desserts, and any other place you can think of!

Tortillas, corn or whole wheat: A flatbread used in Mexican cuisine, which can be wrapped around vegetables, beans, fish, or meats.

Udon noodles: These are Japanese noodles made from whole wheat flour and/or brown-rice flour. Udon can be served hot or cold, and tastes great with tomato sauce. It is shaped like narrow fettuccini. Also see "Pasta," "Soba noodles," "Whole wheat pasta," and "The Whole-Grain and Pasta Story," page 83.

Unsulphured dried fruit: Fruit that is sun-dried or low-heat dried without any sulphur dioxide, which can cause severe reactions in those allergic to it, ranging from nausea to difficulty in breathing.

Vanilla extract: A favorite flavoring for all sorts of sweets. Pure vanilla extract is made from vanilla beans aged in alcohol and is free of sugars, caramel coloring, and other additives. Vanillin is derived from the waste products of the wood-processing industry and we recommend this product never be used. Some manufacturers produce a nonalcoholic, vegetable-oil-based vanilla extract. This and the pure extracts are available in the natural-food stores. (Also look for lemon, orange, and other natural flavors.)

Vinegar: Apple cider and brown-rice vinegars are the two basic culinary vinegars to have on hand. They can be purchased made with organic ingredients.

Water and purified water: See "Water and Purification Systems," page 243.

Whole wheat flour: See "Flour, whole wheat."

Whole wheat pasta: Made from durum wheat, with the bran and germ intact. It has a rich, nutty flavor and is more filling than white or semolina pasta. It is also much more nutritionally beneficial than the refined pastas commonly served. Please see "Pasta," "Soba noodles," "Udon noodles," and "The Whole-Grain and Pasta Story," page 83.

Yogurt: Plain yogurt with living cultures has had the active bacteria added after the milk is pasteurized and the yogurt is made, so they are still active when you eat the yogurt. This type of yogurt provides protein, calcium, and beneficial cultures that inhibit harmful bacteria and promotes better digestion and elimination. The beneficial cultures are lactobacillus bulgaricus, bifidus, lactobacillus acidophilus, and others. Try whole-milk yogurt rather than the low-fat types. Individuals who normally have difficulty digesting milk and milk products may be able to tolerate yogurt better. In recipes, you can substitute yogurt for milk, cream, buttermilk, mayonnaise, or sour cream. We recommend organic yogurt to avoid pesticides and added hormone residues.

Zest, lemon, lime, and orange: When a recipe calls for the zest of a citrus fruit, it is referring to the colored rind. It is preferable to use organic citrus to avoid the anti-mold agents and other chemicals that are sprayed on the skins of citrus fruit before and after harvest. Organic bottled zest can be purchased in the natural-food store.

Friendly Fats

Fats we recommend:

Butter: You will see in our recipes that we do sauté and bake with small amounts of this healthy fat. Butter is a saturated fat, and therefore is stable at relatively high temperatures, and will not break down into PMS-aggravating *trans* fatty acids.

Unsalted or sweet butter has a delicate flavor and since it has no salt, requires the use of fresher cream by the manufacturer, or it will go rancid very quickly. Store several unsalted sticks of butter in the freezer (for up to six months), and one in the refrigerator for daily use (about two weeks). Butter is excellent for baking and light sautéing because it is stable at these higher temperatures and has the best taste. By law, butter has to contain eighty percent butter fat.

We make a special effort to buy only organic butter, which is produced from the cream of cows raised without antibiotics or added hormones. Organic butter can be found in natural-food stores and increasingly in specialty supermarkets. (When considering making the switch from conventionally produced foods to organic foods, this may be the simplest and most effective place to start.) In animals, environmental toxins, antibiotics, and supplemental hormones tend to accumulate in their fatty tissue. Animals raised naturally will have a much lower body concentration of these substances. As butter is composed of the fat component of cow's milk, choosing organic butter is by far the better health choice.

Vegetable and seed oils: A good vegetable oil is one labeled "extra-virgin," or "unrefined" and "expeller pressed." This oil should appear somewhat dark and be close to the color, taste, and smell of the raw ingredient.

Extra-virgin olive oil: This form of olive oil is produced from the first pressing of ripe olives, and is our favorite oil for flavor and health. As it is unrefined, it still contains many nutrients present in the original olive. These include beta-carotene; oil-soluble vitamins such as vitamin E, an antioxidant that acts as a natural preservative in the oil; minerals, such as magnesium; lecithin; essential fatty acids; and phyto-hormones. Perhaps even more importantly, extra-virgin olive oil does not contain *trans* fatty acids. In addition, since olive trees are cultivated according to traditional and more natural methods in most parts of the world, olive oil is also less likely to be contaminated with pesticides.

We do not recommend the other grades of olive oil, including virgin or pure olive oil, which are processed using heat and chemical solvents. Neither do we recommend olive oil labeled "lite." The term "lite" refers to the taste, not the calories. Refined oils, which have little or no taste and are also of lesser quality, are added to olive oil to tone down its full, rich flavor. Don't be fooled. All fats and oils supply the same number of calories, 9 per gram.

Store olive oil in a dark bottle, away from light and heat, and keep only small quantities unrefrigerated for daily use.

Flaxseed oil: At the turn of the century, flaxseed oil was much more commonly used than it is today, but it deserves a revival. Flaxseed oil is nutritious and has a buttery taste that is easy to like. It is exceptionally high in essential fatty acids, composed of about 18 percent linoleic acid and about 57 percent omega-3, linolenic acid. These fats have the special ability of easing menstrual cramping and alleviating many other PMS symptoms, including fluid retention, headaches, and irritability. (Vegetables are another good source of linoleic acid, as are other seeds, and the omega-3 fatty acids are also plentiful in fish and walnuts.)

The essential fatty acids in flaxseed oil break down very quickly and undergo chemical changes when exposed to oxygen, heat, and light. For these reasons, you'll find flaxseed oil in the refrigerator section of your natural-food store, packaged in opaque containers, and sold only in small quantities.

We urge you to treat flaxseed oil with the same tender care in your own kitchen. It's very important to store your flaxseed oil in the refrigerator, even before it's been opened, and to use it up quickly, in about three to six weeks. If you store it in the freezer, you will extend its shelf life to six months. Rather than throwing out oil that has aged, buy only a small bottle each time and regularly replenish your supply. Most importantly, flaxseed oil should *never* be heated. Use it at room temperature when adding it to salad dressings; or if using it as an ingredient in a dish that is served warm, think of flaxseed oil as a condiment and add it once cooking is completed and just before serving.

Unrefined sesame oil: This polyunsaturated oil can be used in cooking. It contains plentiful linoleic acid, an essential fatty acid, and natural preservatives. Unrefined sesame oil is available from natural-food stores.

Dark sesame oil: Especially useful in Asian cooking, dark sesame oil is made from seeds that are roasted before the oil is pressed from them. Since this process begins to break down the oils in the seeds, we prefer not to heat these oils again and only add dark sesame oil as a condiment after a dish is cooked.

Supplement Evening-Primrose, Borage, and Black-Currant Oils

Linoleic acid, found widely in plant foods, will convert to the Series I prostaglandins that reduce menstrual symptoms such as swelling of the extremities, breast tenderness, headaches, and depression. However, as a woman ages, this conversion becomes blocked to some degree. The body has difficulty making an intermediary compound, GLA or gamma-linoleic acid. This blocked conversion can be bypassed using supplemental evening-primrose oil, borage oil, or black-currant oil, all of which contain GLA; many women we speak with say they have noticed a reduction in PMS soon after beginning to supplement with these.

Fats we don't recommend:

Margarine: We have never found the flavor of margarine to be an acceptable replacement for the taste of butter. But the issue with margarine is far more a matter of health. Margarine is a liquid vegetable oil that has been hardened to make it spreadable. After a vegetable oil is processed, it is again exposed to heat and hydrogenated in order to make the oil solid at room temperature. In this process, PMS-promoting *trans* fatty acids are generated as the structure of the oil molecules is altered. (See "Fats and Oils" in the Introduction, page 11.) The production of margarine requires that the oil be heated to a significantly high temperature, from 248° to 410°F (hot enough for deep-frying) for 6 to 8 hours! In addition, nickel and aluminum—metal catalysts—are often used in the process, and these metals can end up in the final product. There is evidence that the intake of aluminum may promote osteoporosis, a concern to women as they age. Many scientists believe that hydrogenated oils may be more damaging than regular saturated fats.

Refined vegetable oils: Many vegetable oils are commonly recommended as being healthy, such as canola and sunflower oils, because they are very low in saturated fats and high in healthy monounsaturated and polyunsaturated fats. These are known to lower the risk of heart disease. However, these oils are normally sold only in their refined form. They lack important nutrients they originally had, but contain *trans* fatty acids. While the word "refined" suggests that the oil has been in some way purified and improved, the refining process actually involves a long string of steps that cause all sorts of vitamins, minerals, and essential fatty acids—as well as flavor and color—to be removed from the oil. Starting with a seed, nut, or bean, these are cleaned and hulled, then flaked and the oil extracted. This oil is then degummed, refined, bleached, deodorized, has preservatives added, and is defoamed so it won't form bubbles in the pan when cooking. To make margarine, this final oil product is then exposed once again to heat and hydrogenated.

Even if a label states that the oil is "unrefined," it must also indicate that it has been cold-pressed, a process that uses only mechanical pressure for extracting oils. Oil that is simply "unrefined" is still extracted using a chemical solvent and then heated to 300°F (150°C) to be distilled.

We have experimented with using unrefined oils, such as corn, canola, and safflower, which are promoted widely in many natural-food stores. Unfortunately, because of their taste and texture we are unable to recommend these also, even though they have been processed in the manner we recommend. For example, safflower oil has a wonderful essential-fatty-acid profile, even better than that of flaxseed oil, but the heavy taste and oily feel of the unrefined and cold-pressed version of safflower oil can ruin a salad dressing or a cake—we speak from experience! Some people also have difficulty digesting these heavier oils. After years of exploration converting recipes from butter to unrefined oils, we have come full circle and have returned to the traditional fats, which we feel are good for you, and taste good.

The Three Kinds of Fats and Oils

Saturated	*Monounsaturated*	
animal fats	almond	macadamia
butter	avocado	olive
lard	cashew	pecan
tropical oils	hazelnut	pistachio

Polyunsaturated Essential Fatty Acids

Omega-3	**Omega-6**
flax oil and seeds	safflower oil
walnuts	sesame oil
other dark leafy greens	soybean oil
organic eggs	sunflower oil
organ meats	pumpkinseed oil
wild game	walnut oil
seaweed	wheat germ oil
fish with high amounts:	almonds
anchovy	hazelnuts
herring	pecans
mackerel	pistachios
roe	walnuts

(Table—Continued)

Omega-3	Omega-6
salmon	sunflower seeds
sardine	pumpkinseeds
trout	sesame seeds
tuna	plant parts other than leaves
fish with moderate amounts:	organic eggs
bluefish	organ meats
oyster	wild game
pompano	whole grains
shark	fowl
striped bass	
swordfish	
turbot	

Plant Foods and Phytohormones

Phytohormones are substances found in plants that have a hormonelike effect in the body. Lignins are one type, found in a variety of plants and seeds. Of all foods, flaxseed oil contains the highest concentrations of lignins, one hundred times more than any plant studied. In descending order, other foods that supply lignins are other seed oils, dried seaweed, legumes, whole grains, vegetables, and fruit. Another type of phytohormone are the isoflavones. These occur in high concentrations in chickpeas, soybeans, and possibly other legumes. Soy flour contains considerably more phytohormones than tofu or soy drinks.

These are the raw materials from which the body constructs various compounds that have a structure similar to estrogen. It has been found that these compounds have the ability to modulate and balance levels of estrogen in the body. When estrogen levels are low, phytohormones can augment the supply, and when estrogen levels are high, phytohormones have an antiestrogenic effect. As symptoms of PMS depend on hormone balance, phytohormones can play a role in achieving this and lessening symptoms.

Other foods in which phytohormones have been identified include lentils, oat bran, kidney beans, wheat, garlic, squash, asparagus, pears, rye, and plums.

Nutrients in Refined Versus Whole Grains

Here is a comparison of the nutrients in refined and whole wheat:

Vitamins and minerals	Nutrients (in mg) in one slice of bread made from enriched white flour	Nutrients (in mg) in one slice of bread made from whole wheat flour
Vitamin B5	.1	.174
Folic acid	9	13
Calcium	20	23
Magnesium	5	18
Phosphorus	22	52
Potassium	24	63
Selenium	6.44	15.5
Zinc	—	.5

The differences between whole grain and refined grain is even more striking in the case of rice:

Vitamins and minerals	Nutrients (in mg) in one cup of enriched white rice	Nutrients (in mg) in one cup of brown rice
Vitamin B6	.3	1
Niacin	6.8	9.2
Vitamin B5	1.26	2.1
Folic acid	20	32
Vitamin E	.7	3
Calcium	47	64
Magnesium	13	172
Manganese	2.1	3.2
Phosphorus	183	432
Potassium	179	420
Selenium	65.1	77.2
Zinc	2.5	3.6

Stocking the Pantry

To help you get started with the purchase of some of the new ingredients we recommend that may not be on your kitchen shelf, we've written the following list:

Beans and Peas

Adzuki, black, black-eyed peas, chickpea, Great Northern, kidney, lentils, lima, navy, pink, pinto, red lentils, split peas.

Whole Grains and Whole-Grain Products

Barley, brown rices, bulgur, couscous, hot and cold cereals, flour, granola, kasha, millet, oatmeal, pancake mix, pastas, rice cakes, quinoa, wild rice, whole-grain breads.

Condiments

Arrowroot, brown-rice and cider vinegars, organic butter, extra-virgin olive oil, flaxseed oil, herbs, herbal sea salt, kuzu, mustard, sea salt, spices.

Miscellaneous

Herbal teas, milk substitutes, nut butters, seaweeds, unsweetened juices.

Brands We Trust

There are many brands of foods we recommend but for some of them we suggest using only certain products. Therefore we have tried to list the specific food items we prefer. The natural-food industry is everchanging and because of this, we suggest you read labels to confirm that the ingredients are of the highest quality and have not altered since publication of this book.

Whole-Grain Pasta, Boxed Grains, Beans, and Mixes

Arrowhead Mills: Red lentils, whole-grain pancake and bread mixes, soup and
   grain mixes
De Boles: A line of organic whole wheat and wheat-free corn pastas
DeCecco: A line of whole wheat pastas
Delverde: A line of whole wheat pastas

Eden Foods: Whole-grain pastas, soba, and udon
Fantastic Foods: Instant soup cups, pilaf, hummus, and other instant bean dishes
Lundberg Farms: The best brown rices and gourmet rice mixes, one-step pilaf and chili mixes, rice cakes, rice pudding mixes
Organica DiSicilia: Organic whole wheat fettuccini and vermicelli pastas
San Gennaro Polenta: Ready-made polenta in a tube
Sobayana: Authentic soba and udon noodles
Vita Spelt: Spelt pasta
Westbrae Natural Foods: Ramen (instant noodles and broth) and other whole-grain pastas

Hot and Cold Cereals

Arrowhead Mills: Whole-grain hot, cold, and puffed cereals
Barbara's: Cold cereals including shredded, flakes, and puffed
Erewhon: Cold cereals including shredded, flakes, and puffed
Good Morning: Granolas
New Morning: Cold cereals and granola

Fats, Oils, and Nut Butters

Alta Dena Certified Dairy: Hormone-free butter
Barleans Organic Oils: Flaxseed and borage oils, expeller pressed and packaged in opaque containers
Colavita: extra-virgin olive oil; available in supermarkets
Flora: Certified organic flaxseed and other quality expeller-pressed oils produced in small amounts to keep the heat and friction at a minimum, and contained in amber glass bottles
Greek Gourmet: organic extra-virgin olive oil
Marathana Natural Foods: Organic raw and roasted nut butters, especially almond
Omega Nutrition, USA: Organic flaxseed oil and other fine-quality cold-pressed oils contained in black bottles
Organic Valley: Certified organic butter and cheeses
Purity Farms: Organic clarified butter or ghee

Herbal Teas, Grain Beverages, and Juices

After the Fall: Unsweetened juices
Bambu: Grain coffee substitute
Cafix: Grain coffee substitute
Celestial Seasonings: Caffeine-free herbal and iced teas
Knudsen & Sons: Organic unsweetened juices

Santa Cruz: Organic unsweetened juices, especially lemon and lime
Traditional Medicinals: Herbal teas designed for various ailments

Condiments, Conserves, and Dried Fruit

Cascadian Farms: Pickles, sauerkraut, relish, organic all-fruit conserves, and organic frozen fruit
Eden Foods: Organic brown-rice and cider vinegars, mustard, miso, soy sauce
Enrico's: Sugar-free barbecue sauce, ketchup, tomato products, and other condiments
Frontier: Salt-free herbs, spices, and pure vanilla extract
Herbamare and Trocomare: Herbal sea salt
Joe's Organic Vegetables and Spices: Certified organic dried vegetables, herbs, and spices
Knudsen & Sons: Organic all-fruit conserves
Lima: Sea salt
Maine Coast: North Atlantic seaweed and seaweed condiments
South River Miso: Chickpea miso
Timbercrest Farms: Unsulphured dried fruits and tomatoes
Westbrae Natural Foods: Sugar-free barbecue sauce, ketchup, and mustard

Milk Substitutes and Yogurt

Hawthorne Valley Farm: Organic yogurt with living cultures
Pacific Foods: Almond milk
Rice Dream: Rice-milk beverages
Seven Stars Farm: Organic yogurt with living cultures
Westbrae Natural Foods: Oat and rice milks

Miscellaneous

Ak-Mak: Whole-wheat sesame crackers
Beyond Gourmet™: Parchment-paper products
Jaclyn's: Whole-wheat bread crumbs
Pamela's Product's, Inc: Wheat-free biscotti, cookies, and baking mixes

Where to Find It

Here is a collection of reliable mail-order sources that offer chemical-free foods:

Beano® Hotline: Call for a free sample. (800) 257-8650.
Broken Arrow Ranch: Wild game. (800) 962-4263.
D'Artagnan: Chicken, turkey, and game. (800) 327-8246.
Diamond Organics: Organic fruits and vegetables. (800) 922-2396.
Flora: Certified organic flaxseed and other quality expeller-pressed oils.
   (800) 498-3610
Rapunzel Pure Organics: Herbal sea salt and teas. (800) 207-2814.
Timber Crest Farms: Unsulphured organic dried fruits, sun-dried tomatoes, fruit
   butters. (707) 433-8251.
Vermont Country Maple Products: Maple syrup. (800) 528-7021.
W & E Allen: Handcrafted maple syrup. (315) 346-6706.
Walnut Acres: A grocery store by mail featuring whole grains and cereals, beans,
   soup mixes, condiments, and more. (800) 433-3998.

A good source for other mail-order foods is:

Green Groceries—A mail-order guide to organic foods, by Jeanne Heifetz
   (HarperCollins, 1992)

Ethnic Menu Choices

Many ethnic restaurants offer nutritious food choices. Each kind has its own specialty. Here is a guide to foods you can order that are on the PMS menu.

Chinese and other Asian foods: steamed fish, vegetables, brown rice, snails,
   shellfish, tofu
Greek: octopus, taramasalta (roe), fish, shellfish, fresh vegetables, beans, stuffed
   vegetables
Indian: dahl (lentils), fresh vegetables, potatoes, vegetarian dishes
Italian: escarole, broccoli rabe, fish, shellfish, baked potatoes
Japanese: miso soup, brown rice, fish, shellfish, tofu, seaweed, vegetables
Latin American: beans, salsa, plantains, salted cod (baccala), root vegetables
   such as battata and melange
Mexican: corn tortillas, beans, salsa, fish, shellfish, fresh vegetables—and hold
   the cheese!
Middle Eastern: bean spreads, baba ganoush (eggplant and vegetables), whole
   wheat pita, shish kebabs

Cookware and Utensils

Owning the right pots and pans and having them accessible eases your tasks in the kitchen. We recommend cookware lined with stainless steel or enamel, although aluminum can be on the outside. We also have a collection of cast-iron and glass cookware. A wok can be handy but is not necessary. If you do buy one, choose a wok made of carbon steel, which is best for heat conduction. Here is a list of some of the more important pieces to own:

1-, 2-, and 3-quart saucepans with lids
8- or 10-inch skillet with lid
10- or 12-inch sauté pan with lid
4-quart pot with lid, for soup and pasta
2-quart Dutch oven
2 cookie sheets
1 baking pan
1 loaf pan or pie plate
1 muffin tin

Knives and Utensils

8-inch chef's knife
Serrated knife
Paring knife
Blender and/or food processor
Colander
Sieve
Vegetable peeler

Sweetness Conversion

Here are a few tips so you can become a pro at dessert-making while still fighting PMS symptoms. You can successfully convert your favorite recipes from white sugar to quality sweeteners by following these guidelines for successful baking:

1. In terms of sweetness, 1 cup of white sugar equals approximately 1 cup of maple syrup. When a dry ingredient is replaced with a liquid one, an equal amount of liquid from the recipe has to be removed, or an equivalent amount of flour can be added.
2. Most standard recipes are too sweet for our tastes, so to compensate we cut

the original amount of white sugar in half. For example, if a recipe begins with 1 cup of sugar, we cut this amount to ½ cup. This converts to ½ cup maple syrup, and the liquid in the recipe is reduced by ½ cup or ½ cup flour is added.

3. Whole-grain flours absorb a little more liquid than white flour. It is helpful to know what the consistency of the original recipe is supposed to be so as to assess whether to remove liquid or add flour. In some recipes there is no liquid to remove, so adding flour is the only choice.

We find it typically takes one or two tries to get the recipe to the correct consistency. Keep notes for the next try—and please know that each trial is usually delicious!

Water and Purification Systems

Water

Clean water is essential to our well-being. The body is about 70 percent water and the normal functioning of all the body systems, organs, and glands, including those involved in the menstrual cycle, are affected by the quality of the water we drink.

In the 1970s, studies conducted by the Environmental Protection Agency found high levels of heavy metals and many chemical contaminants in common household water. Pollutants such as fertilizers, insecticides, and even lead from automobile and factory exhaust were discovered in the lakes and streams. With this research, the government began to set a limit to the types and amounts of chemicals, pesticides, and bacteria permissible in drinking water, and standards were set for radioactivity and turbidity. However, although these standards now exist, they are not enforced nationally. Complicating the picture, new compounds and toxic chemicals continue to be introduced into the water supply, and there are difficulties regulating and testing for these. Certain chemicals are also added to the water supply to counteract the toxins and to make the water more fit to drink. These substances include chlorine, phosphates, sodium aluminates, and lime. Unfortunately, these compounds interfere with the absorption of nutrients and they may also have other toxic side effects.

We think there are many good reasons to make every effort to drink pure water, including carrying a bottle of filtered water in the car when we are away from our own supply at home. You'll also see that in every recipe where water is called for, we recommend using purified water—and we give it the respect it deserves, listing it as an ingredient in its own right.

There are many ways in which you can take charge of the quality of the water you drink. If you rely on bottled waters, be aware that these are not regulated by any governmental agency and that brands vary. There is one brand we do like—Mountain Valley bottled water (see page 245), since it comes in glass bottles. If your water comes from a well, be sure to have it tested regularly for purity. However, most likely you drink and cook using municipal water from the tap, and if this is the case, we strongly recommend using a water purification system to remove toxic substances as well as unwelcome tastes and odors.

Purification Systems

Many filtering systems are designed for countertop use, either by attaching them to the faucet of your kitchen sink or by directly pouring tap water into them. Other units can be installed under the sink or in the basement, and have a separate spigot for the water, leaving your faucet free for washing dishes. Some of these under-counter units purify the water so slowly that a holding tank for the purified water is required to store it. There are three basic types of purification systems and all filters fit into one or more of these classifications. Here is a brief overview.

Solid carbon filters are available for installation attached either to the faucet or under the counter. These install easily and the filters require no electricity to function. The internal filtering cartridge requires replacement once or twice a year. The flow rate is .75 gallons per minute with water available at your tap for immediate use.

Solid carbon filters contain a pre-filter, which removes large particles and rust, and a solid carbon filter that filters a wide variety of heavy metals, chemicals, pesticides, and residues, including DDT and benzene. These filters also contain a micron screen that prevents lead and other toxins from entering the water, but allows particles of healthful minerals, which are relatively small, to pass through.

Granulated carbon filters attach to the faucet or are designed to sit on the top of a holding container. Water from the tap runs through or is poured through a layer of charcoal, which filters out the chlorine and eliminates the chlorine taste. This type of filter needs to be changed about every three weeks since it can only absorb a limited amount of chlorine. In addition, if this type filter is not regularly used and changed, bacterial growth may occur between the chips of charcoal. These units are very similar to fish-tank filters.

Reverse osmosis (RO) can be installed in the basement with a holding tank to store the filtered water, or there is a countertop unit that can be attached to the faucet in the evening to receive and filter water overnight. This water is then stored in plastic containers for later use. No water is available for immediate use at your tap. These units have a pre-filter that removes rust and other large particles, plus a carbon filter that removes many pesticides, chemicals, and residues. There is also a reverse osmosis membrane that removes these same toxins even more thoroughly, but very slowly, wasting a lot of water in the process. The average amount of water produced daily ranges from one and one half to three gallons a day.

Water and Purification Unit Information

Rader and Morrow Health Concepts: (800) 828-9500 (ask for Jane)
Clean Water Concepts, Inc.: P.O. Box 208, South Bound Brook, NJ 08880-0208
  (732) 381-3150
Mountain Valley Water: (800) 643-1501

Resources We Recommend

PMS

Grahm, Judy. *Blood, Bread and Roses—How Menstruation Created the World.* Boston, MA: Beacon Press, 1993.

Lark, Susan M., M.D. *PMS Premenstrual Syndrome Self-Help Book.* Berkeley, CA: Celestial Arts, 1983.

Martorano, Joseph, M.D., and Maureen Motgan, C.S.W., R.N. *Unmasking PMS—The Complete Medical Treatment Plan.* New York: Berkley Books, 1993.

Northrup, Christiane, M.D. *Women's Bodies, Women's Wisdom: Creating Physical and Emotional Health and Healing.* New York: Bantam Books, 1994.

Stepanich, Kisma K. *Sister Moon Lodge—The Power and Mystery of Menstruation.* St. Paul, MN: Llewellyn Publications, 1993.

Nutrition Reference

Appleton, Nancy, Ph.D. *Lick the Sugar Habit.* Garden City, NY: Avery Publishing Group, 1988.

Balch, James F., M.D., and Phyllis A. Balch, C.N.C. *Prescription for Nutritional Healing.* Garden City, NY: Avery Publishing Group, 1990.

Ballantine, Rudolph, M.D. *Diet and Nutrition.* Honesdale, PA: The Himalayan International Institute, 1978.

Dufty, William. *Sugar Blues.* New York: Warner Books, 1975.

Erasmus, Udo, Ph.D. *Fats That Heal—Fats That Kill.* Burnaby, BC, Canada: Alive Books, 1993.

Haas, Elson M., M.D. *Staying Healthy with Nutrition.* Berkeley, CA: Celestial Arts Publishing, 1992.

———. *Staying Healthy with the Seasons.* Berkeley, CA: Celestial Arts Publishing, 1981.

Murray, Michael, N.D., and Joseph Pizzorno, N.D. *Encyclopedia of Natural Medicine.* Revised second edition. Rocklin, CA: Prima Publishing, 1998.

Oski, Frank A., M.D. *Don't Drink Your Milk!* Brushton, NY: TEACH Services, 1992.

Werbach, Melvyn R., M.D. *Nutritional Influences on Illness.* Second Edition. Tarzana, CA: Third Line Press, 1993.

Cooking and Information

Wittenberg, Margaret M. *Experiencing Quality.* Austin, TX: Whole Foods Market, 1987.

De Angelis, Lissa, and Molly Siple. *Recipes for Change.* New York: Dutton, 1996.

PMS Foods to the Rescue!

BEANS

Thiamin (Vitamin B1)
pinto
black
chickpeas
black-eyed peas
soybeans

Riboflavin (Vitamin B2)
pinto
black

Niacin (Vitamin B3)
black
pinto

Pantothenic Acid (Vitamin B5)
all legumes

Pyridoxine (Vitamin B6)
pinto
navy
lima

Folic Acid
cranberry
lentils
mung
adzuki
chickpeas
pinto
pink
lima
Great Northern

black
navy
black-eyed peas
kidney
lupin

Vitamin E
navy

Vitamin K
soybeans
lentils

Boron
soybeans
lentils

Calcium
soybeans
lima
navy
Great Northern
kidney
pinto
chickpeas

Copper
adzuki
soybeans
chickpeas
navy
kidney
lentils
black-eyed peas
Great Northern
cranberry

Iron
black turtle
chickpeas
pinto
navy
soybeans
kidney
lentils
lima

Magnesium
soybeans
white beans
adzuki
lima
Great Northern
cranberry
chickpeas
black
pinto
kidney

Manganese
lima
chickpeas
white beans
soybeans
navy
lentils
pinto
pink
Great Northern
kidney
black-eyed peas

(Beans—Continued)

Phosphorus	**Potassium**	**Zinc**
chickpeas	white beans	adzuki
soybeans	lima	chickpeas
	soybeans	white beans
	pink	black-eyed peas
	black	cranberry
	lentils	soybeans
	kidney	
	split peas	
	adzuki	

FRUIT

Vitamin A
cantaloupe
mango
apricot
persimmon, Japanese
plantain
papaya

Thiamin (Vitamin B1)
grapes
avocado
raisins
pineapple
watermelon
mango

Riboflavin (Vitamin B2)
avocado
peach, dried

Niacin (Vitamin B3)
peach
avocado

Pantothenic Acid (Vitamin B5)
avocado
pomegranate

Pyridoxine (Vitamin B6)
mango
watermelon
banana
avocado
plantain
melon

Folic Acid
avocado

boysenberries
cantaloupe
orange
loganberries
strawberries
papaya

Flavonoids
orange
lemon
lime
grapefruit
black currants
grapes
plums
cherries
apricot
blackberries
papaya
cantaloupe

Vitamin C
papaya
guava
kiwi
lychees
orange
lemon
lime
grapefruit
mango
cantaloupe
watermelon
strawberries
acerola cherries
black currants

Vitamin E
mango

Vitamin K
chayote
avocado
kiwi
strawberries
plums

Boron
apricot, dried
figs, dried
apple
watermelon
pear
peach
grapes
raisins
prunes
dates
cantaloupe
nectarine
apricot
lemon
mango
banana
tangerine

Calcium
figs
cherimoya
papaya
orange
tangerine
boysenberries

Chromium
prunes
grapes
apple
banana

Iron
raisins
peach
mulberries
figs
avocado
pear
currants
boysenberries
prunes

Magnesium
figs
plantain

Manganese
pineapple
banana
loganberries
blackberries
grapes
blueberries

Phosphorus
cherimoya
peach
apricot
raisins
figs
prunes

Potassium
raisins
papaya
plantain
figs
black currants
cantaloupe
apricot
avocado
banana

GRAINS

Thiamin (*Vitamin B1*)
whole rye
wild rice
whole wheat
millet
buckwheat
bulgur
couscous, whole wheat
brown rice

Riboflavin (*Vitamin B2*)
wild rice
millet
whole wheat

Niacin (*Vitamin B3*)
whole wheat
brown rice
whole barley
bulgur
couscous, whole wheat
millet

**Pantothenic Acid
    (*Vitamin B5*)**
all whole grains

Pyridoxine (*Vitamin B6*)
brown rice
whole wheat
whole rye
bulgur
couscous, whole wheat

Folic Acid
whole wheat
whole barley
brown rice

Flavonoids
buckwheat

Vitamin E
millet
whole oat
whole wheat
cornmeal

Boron
whole rye
millet
buckwheat
cornmeal
whole barley
whole oat

Calcium
cornmeal
whole wheat
brown rice

Chromium
whole wheat
brown rice
whole oats

Iron
millet
brown rice
wild rice
whole rye
buckwheat
whole wheat

Magnesium
buckwheat
whole wheat

cornmeal
bulgur
couscous, whole wheat
whole rye
millet
brown rice
quinoa

Manganese
whole wheat
brown rice
buckwheat
whole rye
whole oat

Phosphorus
brown rice
cornmeal
whole wheat
whole oat
whole rye
quinoa

Potassium
whole rye
millet
buckwheat
whole barley

Selenium
whole wheat
brown rice

Zinc
brown rice
whole wheat
cornmeal

MEAT

Vitamin A
beef liver

Thiamin (Vitamin B1)
pork
liver
venison

Riboflavin (Vitamin B2)
liver
kidney
caribou
antelope
goat
venison

Niacin (Vitamin B3)
liver
beef
lamb
rabbit
venison

**Pantothenic Acid
  (Vitamin B5)**
beef liver
caribou
kidney

Pyridoxine (Vitamin B6)
pheasant
turkey
chicken
duck
quail

**Vitamin B12
  (Cobalamin)**
liver

kidney
beef
pork
lamb
rabbit
caribou
tongue

Folic Acid
liver
beef
pork
lamb

Vitamin C
liver

Vitamin D
liver

Vitamin E
lamb
organ meats

Vitamin K
beef liver
beef

Boron
kidney

Chromium
liver
beef

Copper
liver
kidney

Iodine
liver

Iron
liver
venison
quail
beef
pork
lamb
heart
tongue
kidney
caribou

Phosphorus
pork
beef
venison
liver

Potassium
beef
pork
lamb

Selenium
chicken
turkey

Zinc
liver
beef
beefalo
goat
caribou
lamb
tongue

NUTS

Thiamin (Vitamin B1)
Brazil nut
pine nut
pistachio
pecan
hazelnut
cashew

Riboflavin (Vitamin B2)
almond
hazelnut
chestnut
cashew

Niacin (Vitamin B3)
peanut
almond

Pyridoxine (Vitamin B6)
walnut
hazelnut
peanut
chestnut

Folic Acid
pistachio

Vitamin E
almond
Brazil nut
hazelnut
peanut

Vitamin K
pistachio

Boron
almond
hazelnut
peanut
walnut
pecan

Calcium
hazelnut
Brazil nut
almond

Copper
cashew
Brazil nut
hazelnut
pistachio
walnut
almond

Iron
pistachio
almond
cashew
Brazil nut
hazelnut

Magnesium
cashew
Brazil nut
walnut
almond

Manganese
Brazil nut
chestnut
hazelnut
almond
peanut
walnut
pine nut
pecan

Phosphorus
Brazil nut
peanut
almond
cashew
pistachio
walnut

Potassium
pistachio
almond
peanut
Brazil nut
hazelnut

Selenium
Brazil nut

Zinc
Brazil nut
cashew
pecan
peanut

OILS

Vitamin A
fish liver

Vitamin E
sunflower
almond
peanut
safflower
sesame
soybean
olive
flax
wheat germ

Vitamin K
safflower
fish liver
olive

POULTRY

Vitamin A
egg
chicken liver

Thiamin (Vitamin B1)
duck
quail

Riboflavin (Vitamin B2)
chicken, dark meat
liver
heart

Niacin (Vitamin B3)
chicken
turkey
pheasant
quail
liver

**Pantothenic Acid
   (Vitamin B5)**
liver
chicken
heart
goose

Pyridoxine (Vitamin B6)
pheasant
turkey
chicken
duck
quail

**Vitamin B12
   (Cobalamin)**
liver
heart

Folic Acid
liver
turkey
chicken
quail
egg

Vitamin D
egg yolk

Vitamin E
egg

Vitamin K
egg yolk

Chromium
turkey

Iodine
egg

Iron
egg
heart
liver
duck

Magnesium
egg yolk

Phosphorus
goose
chicken
turkey
duck
egg
pheasant

Selenium
chicken
turkey

Zinc
chicken
duck
pheasant
turkey
egg
heart

SEAFOOD

Thiamin (Vitamin B1)
lobster
trout
oysters
tuna
catfish

Riboflavin (Vitamin B2)
clams
salmon
mackerel
oysters
trout
herring

Niacin (Vitamin B3)
tuna
swordfish
mackerel
shad
sturgeon
eel
salmon
trout
halibut
oysters
shrimp
sardines

**Pantothenic Acid
(Vitamin B5)**
bluefish
abalone
trout
salmon
cod

Pyridoxine (Vitamin B6)
tuna

trout
salmon
bluefish
octopus

**Vitamin B12
(Cobalamin)**
clams
octopus
oysters
mussels
mackerel
herring
tuna
crabs
eel
snails
trout
salmon
striped bass

Folic Acid
trout
oysters
tuna

Vitamin C
oysters

Vitamin D
kippers
mackerel
salmon
catfish
oysters
tuna
sardines
shrimp
perch

herring
cod
flounder
sole
halibut

Vitamin E
shrimp
haddock
mackerel
herring
salmon
oysters
perch

Vitamin K
abalone

Boron
shrimp

Calcium
sardine, with bones
mackerel, with bones
shrimp
salmon, with bones
perch
crabs
soft-shell crabs
clams
oysters

Chromium
clams
haddock

Copper
oysters
squid

mussels
clams
crabs
octopus
crayfish

Iodine
haddock
perch
salmon
tuna
sole
oysters
shrimp

Iron
clams
oysters
tuna
snails
abalone
shrimp
caviar
octopus
mussels

Magnesium
shrimp
oysters
halibut
mackerel

Manganese
mussels
clams
bass
trout
pike
perch
smelt
oysters

Phosphorus
mackerel
lobster
bluefish
crabs
carp
pollock
catfish
salmon
shad
flounder

Potassium
dried salt cod
flounder
trout
halibut
grouper
pompano
octopus
clams
salmon

Selenium
shrimp
smelt
clams
lobsters
crabs
scallops
cod
flatfish
tuna
oysters
salmon
mackerel
flounder
sole
perch
haddock

Zinc
oysters
crabs
lobsters
herring

SEEDS

Thiamin (Vitamin B1)
sunflower
flax
sesame

Riboflavin (Vitamin B2)
pumpkinseed
squash
sunflower

Niacin (Vitamin B3)
sunflower

**Pantothenic Acid
   (Vitamin B5)**
sunflower

Pyridoxine (Vitamin B6)
sunflower
flax

Vitamin E
sunflower

Boron
flax

Calcium
sesame

Copper
sunflower
sesame
pumpkinseed

Iron
pumpkinseed
sunflower
sesame

Magnesium
pumpkinseed
squash
watermelon
sesame
sunflower
flax

Manganese
sunflower
pumpkinseed

Phosphorus
pumpkinseed
sunflower
sesame

Potassium
sunflower
sesame

Selenium
sesame
sunflower

Zinc
pumpkinseed
sesame
sunflower

VEGETABLES

Vitamin A
sweet potatoes
yams
carrots
winter squash
  butternut
  acorn
  buttercup
  Hubbard
pumpkin
lamb's-quarters
shallots
dark leafy greens
  spinach
  dandelion
  turnips
  kale
  collards
  beet greens
  mustard
  chicory
red peppers
taro
bok choy
scallions
parsley
broccoli
asparagus

Thiamin (Vitamin B1)
potatoes
peas, green
Jerusalem artichoke
nori seaweed
fresh corn
okra

Riboflavin (Vitamin B2)
yams

mushrooms
winter squash
  butternut
  acorn
  buttercup
  Hubbard
kombu
nori

Niacin (Vitamin B3)
mushrooms
potatoes
asparagus
peas, green
corn, fresh
Jerusalem artichokes
broccoli
summer squash
nori
hiziki

**Pantothenic Acid
(Vitamin B5)**
shiitake mushrooms

Pyridoxine (Vitamin B6)
spinach
broccoli
bok choy
potatoes

Folic Acid
asparagus
beets
soybean sprouts
turnip greens
peas, green
artichokes
okra

spinach
leeks
yard-long beans
mustard greens
lentil sprouts

Flavonoids
green peppers
tomatoes
broccoli

Vitamin C
red peppers
broccoli
Brussels sprouts
green peppers
kohlrabi
snow peas
mustard greens
sweet potatoes
cabbage
kale
lamb's-quarters
alfalfa sprouts
tomatoes
cassava root
potatoes
parsley

Vitamin D
shiitake mushrooms,
  dried
button mushrooms

Vitamin E
sweet potatoes
asparagus
avocados
cucumbers
kale

(Vegetables—Continued)

collards
seaweed
cabbage

Vitamin K
cauliflower
watercress
asparagus
broccoli
Brussels sprouts
kale
spinach
Swiss chard
cabbage
turnip greens
endives
mustard greens
broccoli
watercress
lettuce
peas, green
tomatoes
green beans
kelp
parsley
snow peas
artichokes
green peppers
cucumbers
potatoes
celery

Boron
dark leafy greens
dandelions
spinach
potatoes
broccoli
parsley

radishes, white
beets
artichokes
peas, green
shallots
cabbage
carrots
onions
pumpkin
asparagus
leeks

Calcium
dark leafy greens:
    lamb's-quarters
    turnip greens
    chicory
    bok choy
    collards
    dandelions
    mustard
    kale
    cabbage
kelp
okra
acorn squash
butternut squash
rutabaga
carrots
artichokes
agar-agar

Chromium
mushrooms
beets
asparagus
seaweed
potatoes
broccoli

green beans
tomatoes

Copper
potatoes
avocados
shiitake mushrooms,
    dried

Iodine
kelp
spinach
potatoes
broccoli
mushrooms
asparagus

Iron
Jerusalem artichokes
parsley
leeks
peas
artichokes
scallions
spinach
beets
kuzu
seaweed
    agar-agar
    dulse
    wakame

Magnesium
spinach
beets and beet greens
broccoli
potatoes with skin
avocados

(Vegetables—Continued)

Manganese
collards
okra
peas
seaweed

Potassium
potatoes
Swiss chard
beet greens
spinach
seaweed
tomatoes, dried
cassava root

Selenium
carrots
cabbage
mushrooms
cauliflower
fresh corn
potatoes
green beans
garlic
seaweed

Zinc
fresh corn
mushrooms
seaweed

MISCELLANEOUS FOODS

Vitamin A
butter

Thiamin (Vitamin B1)
tahini

Riboflavin (Vitamin B2)
yogurt
miso

Niacin (Vitamin B3)
miso

Pyridoxine (Vitamin B6)
blackstrap molasses

**Vitamin B12
 (Cobalamin)**
yogurt

Folic Acid
beer

Flavonoids
rose hips

Vitamin C
rose hips
sauerkraut

Vitamin D
sunshine

Vitamin E
blackstrap molasses

Vitamin K
blackstrap molasses
miso
pickle

Boron
honey
cinnamon
cider
beer

Calcium
blackstrap molasses
yogurt, whole, plain
goat cheese
sesame butter
tofu
tempeh

Chromium
beer
maple syrup

Copper
blackstrap molasses
chocolate, baker's
sesame butter
cashew butter
miso
natto

Iodine
yogurt, whole, plain

Iron
blackstrap molasses
natto
sesame butter

Magnesium
blackstrap molasses
chocolate, bitter
sunflower-seed butter
natto
tahini
cashew butter
tofu

Manganese
chocolate, bitter
carob
natto
maple syrup
tempeh
tofu
miso

Phosphorus
butter
brewer's yeast
sheep cheese
goat cheese

Potassium
sauerkraut
pickle
natto

Selenium
blackstrap molasses

Zinc
sauerkraut
miso

INDEX

Index